The Ride

New Zealand
and the Long Road Back to Health

Judson Kempton Main

Maingalaxy Consulting
1740H Dell Range Boulevard
Suite 417
Cheyenne, WY 82009
jmain@maingalaxyconsulting.com

Ordering Information:
Quantity sales. Special discounts are available on quantity purchases by corporations, associations, and others. For details, contact the author.

Formatted, edited, and reviewed for publication by Suzette Vaughn. She was patient and absolutely invaluable to the success of this book.
Edited by Grammargal (find her on Fivver). Thanks to her for her excellent work.

Printed in the United States of America

First edition

Hardcover: 978-1-7333324-2-2
Paperback: 978-1-7333324-0-8
Kindle Edition: 978-1-7333324-1-5

10 9 8 7 6 5 4 3 2 1

Dedication

To my Sifu and friend Tim Sheehan.
Your inspiration on how to live and how to be made this book possible.

Acknowledgments

I'd like to thank F. Scot Anderson, my best-buddy and mentor, for giving me the opportunity to learn Unix, for bringing me on to your security team, and watching out for me over the years through some really tough times. Your advice and friendship have meant the world to me.

I'd also like to thank my mother and sister and brother-in-law, all of whom supported me in bad times, and encouraged me in good.

To Todd Nyholm, good friend and great rolfer, who is still recovering from health concerns far worse than mine, who's been an inspiration, and has really helped me get through this mess.

To Jennifer Zygnut for being a good friend, and her help and support for moving this book down the road.

To Jillianne Wilkinson, a good friend, who brings light to the dark, and brought joy to a great friend.

I have a great group of friends whom also should recognized for their inspiration as well: James Childress, Sarah Burnett, Carl Nesse, Travis Krause, Andrea Pinedo, and Kirk Trojovsky.

And finally, Dr. Bill Billica. Bless you, sir, for your knowledge, your approaches, and your self. You do a world of good for many people, improving our lives tremendously, and it just doesn't get any better than that.

Table of Contents

Table of Figures

Foreword

If just one person who reads this book gets cured of Lyme disease or any of its co-infections, then the goal of this book has been achieved.

The Ride

New Zealand
and the Long Road Back to Health

Judson Kempton Main

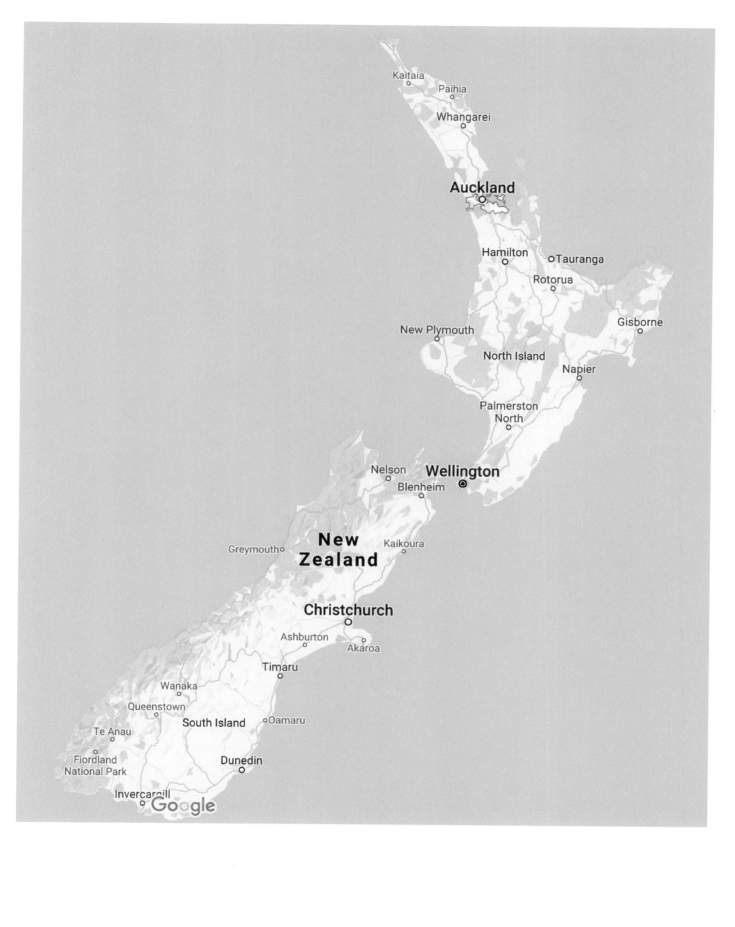

Chapter One - The Beginning

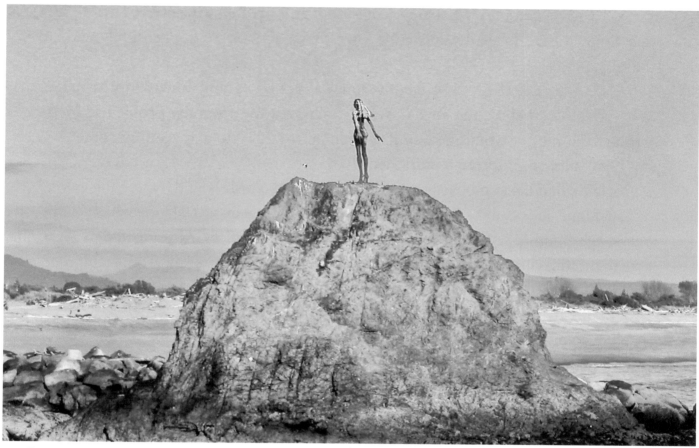

Figure 1 - Statue at the entrance to Whakatane harbor

It was back in 2002, and I was sitting on a ferry at the wharf of the little town of Whakatane (Fa-ka-ta-ni) in New Zealand, waiting to head out to a small volcano a few miles north of the coast, when the song "Strong" by Robbie Williams started playing, and I realized for the first time in months I felt good.

And that meant something was really, *really* wrong.

I had been working for two years at a dot-com, a work environment more dysfunctional and stressful than any I'd experienced before. Hell, after one year I had three bags under each eye and a stress attack that landed me in the hospital. Even a week at a resort south of Cancun with my girlfriend did little to fix the damage.

So after another long year, I quit, broke up with my girlfriend, sold a car, and with the cash flew to Auckland, New Zealand, bought a bike, and started riding. I was forty pounds overweight, way out of shape, with a kneecap that was, once again, trying to dislocate itself. I was all kinds of a mess.

After eight weeks of brutal rides over long distances, into the wind and uphill both ways, I had settled into Whakatane, burnt out and tired, but twenty pounds lighter and able to jog through the hills above the town for an hour or so. Yet I still felt awful, every day.

Why? Why did I feel so bad all the time? What was going on with my knee (again)? Why couldn't I handle the stress? Was I running away from my problems? What was wrong with me? It would take until December of 2017 to start getting some answers, but I had a lot to go through until then.

New Zealand is composed of three islands: The North Island, where the capital city of Auckland is located, the South Island, and then Stewart Island, which is directly below the South Island. New Zealand is fifteen hundred miles southeast of Australia, and about thirty-six degrees south latitude. Yes, the climate is just wonderful: moderate temps all year round, as the Pacific is still fairly warm. Humans are still outnumbered fifty to one by sheep, and the sun is upside down in the sky.

The country is fairly safe, compared to Australia. The Moa, a seven-foot tall bird/predator, is long extinct. There are no cougars, or panthers, or lions, or tigers, or bears. There are relatively few things that can kill you should you go astray, you know, other than a supervolcano, and then we're all ash.

I mean, Australia is crazy. It's as if two scientists, part of some long-lost ancient high civilization, decided to get into a game of "who can create the most poisonous, dangerous, scary looking thing on the planet" just because they could.

Anyway, I was told that Auckland has the largest percentage of boat ownership of any city in the world, and I believe it. It's a big city, with a population of around 1.6 million. It also has half the population of the whole country. Marinas were everywhere, as were harbors, inlets, and all kinds of little places to hide within the seven old volcanos that surround the bays.

The indigenous people (since about 700 years ago) are the Maori, who are Polynesian in origin. Good folk, and through wise legal representation throughout the years of the British invasions have retained ownership of a large portion of the land.

Before them, nobody knows who was there, though some reddish human hairs were found in a cave which sent some into a tizzy, and in 1875 there was a news report of the discovery of giant skeletons (well, seven feet tall), and again in later years, but these have since been hushed up for who knows what reason. I think it's always good to have a bit of mystery; it adds to the flavor.

In addition to the Maori and the English, there were the Scots, who migrated to the South Island and created Dunedin and Invercargill, among other cities. The former is a play on Edinburgh, the latter probably translates to something dirty. ☺

The North Island is in the shape of a four-armed starfish, with the top arm being the longest, extending north by northwest into the subtropics, with the other three being rather stubby. The South Island is located somewhat west of the North and is runs northeast to southwest. One travels laterally between the islands via ferry, along Cook's Strait which is known for huge currents and gigantic, ship-sucking whirlpools, plus the occasional thirty- to forty-foot wave.

I had bought my bicycle online—an Avanti mountain bike with full panniers and plenty of gears–and picked it up in Auckland, but I noticed quickly while riding around the city that my instincts were all wrong, as everyone drives on the wrong side of the road. I kept looking left when I should have been looking right. I rode a bit around Auckland anyway, staying off the roads as much as possible, just getting used to the bike.

I had arrived in the fall (for them, early spring for me) and needed to get to the South Island to start my ride before it turned too cold. An overnight train took me to Wellington, which went by fine, but the ride from the train station over to the ferry terminal was hair-raising. It's a three-kilometer section of road with no shoulder, no room, nowhere to go, and cars flying by you so close you could touch their doors.

I had another cyclist following behind me, both of us racing along trying to put this section behind us and get to safety. Suddenly, from the right, embedded in the road, came railroad tracks at a very narrow angle to our direction. This is death to all two-wheeled vehicles, and the little channels were just wide enough to catch a bicycle's tires. With traffic whizzing by I nonetheless took a steep-angled approach and made it across without bloodshed, but my follower did not. I don't know what happened—maybe she was concentrating on traffic—but her front wheel got caught and up and over she went, doing a face-plant on the pavement. Fortunately the minivan following us stopped in time.

She was very shaken, with a cut above the nose and a bruised mouth. In her own words, it was her first crash in over five thousand kilometers of riding. I felt really, really bad (and still do), as there was a frontage road off to my left, with no tracks and far few cars, and I should had led us there.

Fortunately, a fellow stopped to help and had a med kit handy. I pulled our rigs off onto the frontage road while she recovered, and eventually, an ambulance showed up and gave her a ride over to her destination, in this case a "backpackers." Backpackers, aka hostels, are cheap places to stay offering shared accommodations, usually for wandering college students, or anyone wanting to meet up with fellow travelers.

The mechanic at the garage we had all gathered in front of said that fifteen to twenty bicyclists do face-plants at that exact location each year. One got hit and had to be taken to the hospital. The city council had been told, several times, of the problems with those tracks, but nothing had been done yet. (Of course, this is now seventeen years ago, so let's cross our fingers and hope it's since been handled.)

The ferry brought me over to the little town of Picton on the South Island. Once there I did a short ride and realized quickly that (1) it was a long way to the next town, and (2) I was way out of shape for that kind of distance. Remember these words: everywhere you go in New Zealand there's a thousand-foot climb, and only one way to get there from here. So I took a bus down to Christchurch and finally started my ride.

Chapter Two - A Brief History

I grew up in Setauket, Long Island, New York, in the middle of an oak and maple forest on the North Shore, about a quarter mile as the crow flies from the Long Island Sound, but I was born in California. We had moved when I was only five when my dad got a job as a professor of history at Stony Brook University. I was a happy, athletic, well-adjusted little ball of trouble, as most young boys are, until the age of seven, when things suddenly changed: I became a withdrawn, depressed, uncoordinated, unathletic mess. I had no idea why. Hell, my best guess was that I was all heartbroken when my girlfriend broke up with me. (Let's hear it for puppy love!)

Yeah, I had a girlfriend at the age of six. Very pretty half-Chinese, half-Japanese girl; her dad had won a Nobel Prize in physics. It took until my senior year in high school to have the guts to ask her out again, and while she graciously agreed and we had a nice evening, there was nothing there.

Anyway, back in elementary school, almost every day I left my lunch on the front hall table, driving my mom crazy, as she had to drive to the school to get it to me. I was told this was inherited—a family trait. I sure had it bad. There's a family story I might as well tell now. . .

My dad's father was a professor at the University of Wisconsin, Madison. He was so absent-minded that one day he drove his car into town, then after a day of classes walked back home to find it missing. After some investigation, the local constabulary called his wife back, saying, "Dorothy, he's done it again!"

I still can't remember much of second, third, or fourth grade. Sometime in my mid-thirties I did remember that once, back in third grade, I dragged my desk up to the front of the class right next to the teacher and proceeded to build a wall with some cardboard boxes between myself and the rest of the class. The teacher had called my mom about this incident, but they didn't know what to do. There's no way they could have known what was wrong anyway.

I became the strikeout king of little league, which was weird because when I was younger, I could hit everything. It certainly didn't help my self-esteem. I kept playing, though, God knows why, and while I don't remember most of it, there was one game when I got a hit off a friend - boy was he pissed!

I couldn't run fast (though was quick), was kind of short, couldn't jump, didn't float, couldn't swim much at all, so sport options were limited to ping-pong and tennis. Eventually I got pretty good at the latter, though a knee injury in high school just after I'd made varsity put a quick end to any dreams there. The knee continues to be a problem to this day, though it appears the root cause has finally been discovered.

My friends and I grew up in a time when parents allowed their children to disappear for the entire day, only expecting them back around dinner time. If you got hurt, you brushed it off and kept going. If you crashed on your bike (we rode them everywhere), you didn't cry, because you didn't want your friends to see you cry. Very good training for life.

We learned to invent games on our own—cops and robbers, mostly, and occasionally took our tents into the woods and spent the night. There wasn't a lot of traffic: this area wasn't on the way to anywhere else, and there was only one road along which cars tended to speed so we knew to be careful there. Sidewalks were rare, so again, you rode or walked on the street.

Mostly we rode; to the beach, through the woods, down to the mill ponds, to the deli, and anywhere else. Yes, no helmets, no lights, no nothing. In all the time growing up I only heard of one bicycle death: a fellow on what we called back then a "10-speed" (they call 'em road bikes now), at a known dangerous intersection, was trying to take a left turn and got hit hard by a car. My family came upon the accident just after it happened; not even the police were on the scene yet. My brother got out to take a closer look and said he knew the guy.

And the police were cool. That's right, cool. They weren't out to be assholes, and the laws hadn't changed to force them to be assholes. They were out to look after the citizenry and take care of them when issues arose.

My brother (older by four years) went through a time of hard drinking in his early teen years. One morning I went downstairs to find him on the couch, his face all scratched up. Turns out after drinking with friends and walking back home, he blacked out and fell into some thorny bushes. The cops picked him up and delivered him home, with only a stern warning to the parents. No tickets, no juvenile detention, no weird drugs. My brother turned out wonderful in the end, thankyouverymuch.

There were no street lights in the neighborhoods, and it could get very, *very* dark at night, which was just *amazing*. One of my favorite memories is of riding my bike along West Meadow Road, in a dark so dark I couldn't see the road in front of me. It was the height of summer, humid and still; and the crickets were singing. Doesn't get any better than that.

By high school I had many questions. Why am I always depressed? I hated myself, for a number of reasons. Why can't I hit a baseball to save my life? Why do I feel separated from everyone else? What is the deal with my memory? (Was it really just inherited?) Why am I not allowed to defend myself?

This last one was odd indeed: the older brother of a friend of mine thought it was "cool" to set him up in fights against me. I refused to defend myself, which is just all kinds of odd. Basic survival behavior 101: defend yourself. This is an instinct so natural that to not do so is almost a psychotic response. I worked it out eventually, with him, and with myself. What's funny and sad is that I thought all of this was normal. Perspective is indeed a bitch.

Chapter Three - Starting the Ride

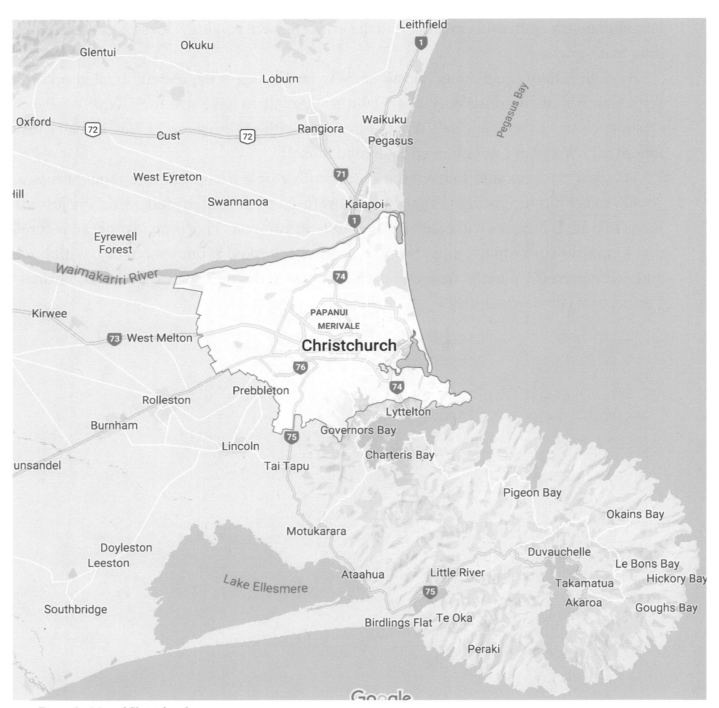

Figure 2 - Map of Christchurch

Christchurch is the high-tech center of New Zealand. Located on the east coast of the South Island, it's also a fisherman's paradise, as there's a deep-sea shelf a ways out over which all kinds of schools of fish congregate, attracting whales, dolphins, and all manner of other kinds of predator and prey.

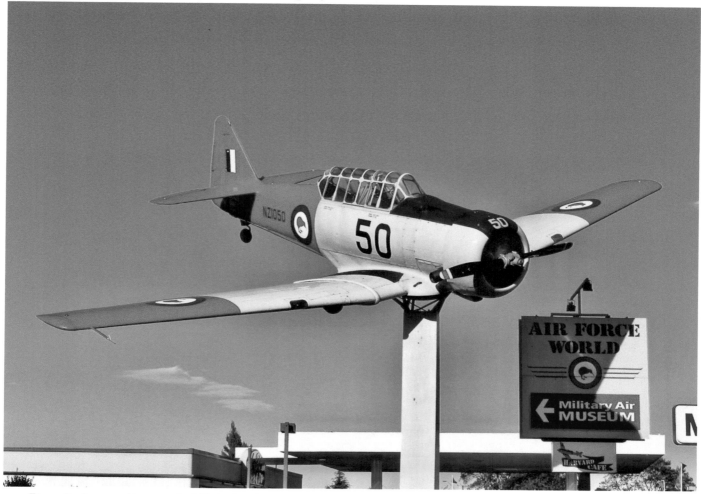

Figure 3 - Japanese Zero, south of Christchurch

I didn't get many pics of the area; I was at this time too determined to get moving. I was bound for Dunedin, where a bunch of Scots had settled and even started up a whiskey distillery (making it high on my list of places to visit). That little city was 361 kilometers away, about 216 miles.

They aren't bike friendly in this country. They drive fast, there's often no shoulder (especially through the hills and mountains), and on bridges there can be no room to maneuver. Thankfully there are not a lot of cars, so you time your "run" past the danger during the gaps in traffic.

The rides are long, and hard. My first was "only" forty-eight kilometers (so say my notes of this trip!). Now when you're out of shape, on a bike that weighs, including gear, around thirty-five pounds, and the average distance between towns is going to be like this, days off to recuperate are frequent. It is, of course, worse when the wind kicks up. On this run it was strong, and from the southwest—into my right-front quarter.

This area of the country is just like Colorado, with farms, sheep, cattle, and bare-looking hills in the distance. Much of the east side of the South Island is like this: dry, relatively barren, but with beautiful, clear beaches. A huge spine of mountains that span the west-center of the island from north to south blocks the rain.

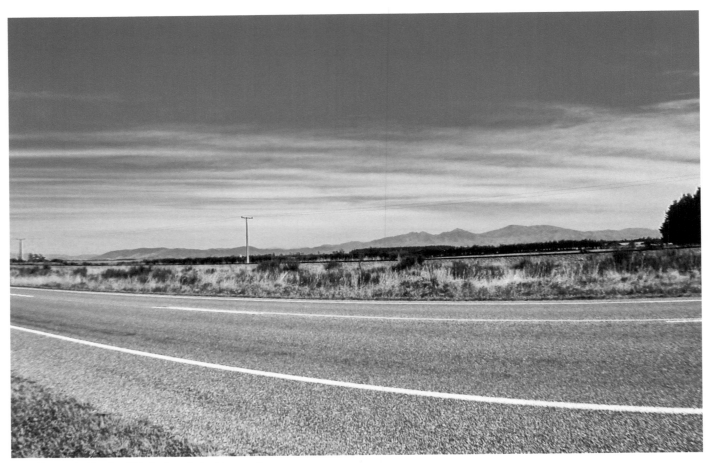

Figure 4 - South of Christchurch, looking west

I was here, on my bike, on a mission: to work off the tremendous stress from a job that started as a sales engineering job, changing quickly to VP of Support Services within six weeks of joining the firm! Every week I was given a new department to manage: Support, Documentation, Training . . .

Well it turned out the completely spineless CTO, one of the company founders, didn't have the guts just to fire the current guy, and didn't even tell me there *existed* another guy. He of course was giving instructions to his now former employees as if nothing had happened. So I would give guidance to our two Documentation people, and they would get a different set from the other fellow.

Eventually the other guy was let go, but this kind of other crap would continue for my entire tenure. I'd go to work, work as hard and fast as I possibly could to manage a complete nightmare, then go home to a girlfriend who wanted all of my attention.

Within a year I had my first stress attack. I lasted another year in a lesser position, gutting it out, but I had burned myself out. I should have quit earlier. Had I known I'd been fighting a *major friggin' disease* for all of my life, I would have.

Perspective is the hardest thing to grasp of all, and I just thought all of my problems were normal. "Gutting it out" is what us men do: for family, for friends, for employees. It's normal, healthy, instinctive male behavior, and I had all of that, plus a big stubborn streak to boot. But I also had a feeling all my life that deep down, wherever I went, there I was, and there was something very wrong too; I just didn't know what. I thought it was me, my problem, a weakness in my character, something that was all my fault. Lords knows some of that was true, just not all of it.

Forty-eight kilometers down the road from Christchurch I finished my first big ride at the little town of Rakaia, where for only NZ$18 (about US$9 back then) I rented a dinky little one-room cabin and collapsed.

The next day I did a twenty-eight kilometer ride (about seventeen miles) and ended up in Ashburton and spoiled myself: for NZ$90 I got a hotel room with a jacuzzi, kitchen, "plunger" (which is a French press), couple of cookies, small sewing kit, thing for buffing up good shoes, hair dryer, ironing board, and more. Very nice, and the jacuzzi about saved me. (You should know that all hotel rooms in New Zealand have small fridges, microwaves, pots, dishes, silverware, cups, coffeemakers, etc.)

The next day I went a little crazy and completed an eighty-kilometer ride into Timaru. Of course there had to be some small hills along the way which I barely made up and over. One time while panting and puffing hard I heard a bird sing, "How dry I am," and laughed and thought to myself, "*That* should be the national bird of this country." Pubs outnumber churches by a long shot and God forbid if you don't follow the New Zealand All Blacks rugby team.

Rugby is kind of a poor man's football. ☺ (I got teased by the locals about NFL players, "Why are they always patting each other on the butts?" so this is my pay-back.) But those rugby players are TOUGH. They play without pads or helmets yet seem to have a lot less injuries.

Timaru is a very beautiful little seaside resort, with a great beach for swimming. The day's ride had taken me over five and a half hours; I was absolutely exhausted, and my legs were shot. I was getting better at riding, though: my pedaling was more circular, and I was now learning to both push and pull. This alone had increased my speed by almost 5k per hour. Dunedin was still 200k away with a small mountain guarding the northern approach. It was going to be tough.

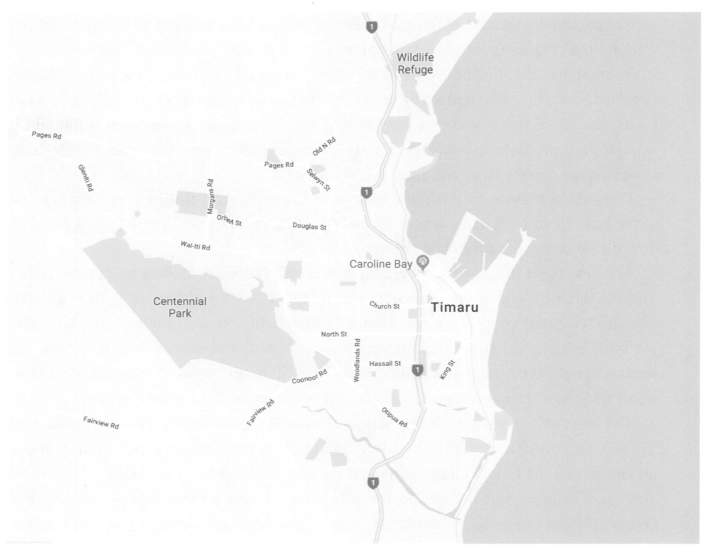

Figure 5 - Map of Timaru - South of Christchurch on the way to Dunedin

Was this bike ride me running away from a challenge again? This feeling inside had given me a fight or flight feeling, and I had developed the habit of the latter, running away from problems, instead of dealing with them and fighting hard. I had run away before: from a good friend back in ninth grade, and from a situation with a company called Fibreview among others.

With the friend, for example, my family had moved to Walla Walla, Washington for a year when I was in ninth grade, and I made some new friends, especially one fellow with whom I hung out with a lot. But for whatever reason, after we moved back, I didn't want to talk to him or any of the friends I had made there. He wasn't the only one I did that to. I guess in some way different people reminded me how much I didn't like some aspect of myself.

In 1984, desperate to change and looking for answers, I found one of the premier martial arts school in country, based out of Greeley, Colorado, and slowly started to get myself sorted out, physically, emotionally, and mentally. The school was all that I needed and more. Hell, still is.

I joined Fiberview a couple years later, when I was doing temporary work here and there through various agencies and had become friends with the owner who hired me on to this, his newest venture. But I hit a crossroads when a critical product delivery meant working non-stop into the wee hours of the morning for a week, which would have meant I'd miss my martial arts classes, and my Sifu was already on my ass for missing some sessions. The owner still doesn't know that I just didn't have the stamina to do both or even just for him during that crunch time, but again, I didn't know it at the time. Of course I chose to attend my classes, but to this day I have regrets and wish I had at least *tried* to do both.

A few years later, though, I quit my martial arts school because I had hit an impasse, personally and professionally, and was screwing up both. I couldn't gain traction in any field, couldn't get my love life straight, couldn't figure out how to just buckle down, work really hard, and move thing forward.

After more odd jobs, including life as a taxicab driver, I moved to northern Virginia where I stayed with my sister and brother-in-law for a bit while on my way to North Carolina. My destination was the Research Triangle Park in the middle of Raleigh, Durham, and Chapel Hill. But my car broke down, and in bits and pieces it ended up taking all of my cash just to keep it running, leaving me stranded in McLean.

So I joined a temp agency just to get a job, any job, to refill the coffers. The first gig I got was answering phone calls from little old ladies in the Midwest for the Pat Buchanan presidential campaign. Seriously. I lasted two days and then pleaded with the home office, "No mas!"

The next gig was as a secretary (oh, excuse me, "executive assistant") for someone who had no work for me to do, leaving me to sit at a desk twiddling my thumbs all day. This much has always been true: if you want to drive me crazy, give me nothing to do. (Hey, that rhymes!) So I harassed the poor woman for work until she finally pawned me off onto another group that was coordinating the IRS GO-ELF (online electronic tax filing) effort. This was a valiant attempt by all those involved, but this was back in 1996, and the Internet hadn't matured enough to make it happen, and the project eventually failed.

But I got pretty good at HTML (the programming language behind most web pages), which I used for creating all of the various tax forms. Then my mentor-to-be and future best buddy Scot Anderson pulled me onto his cybersecurity team and threw me into a closet full of Hewlett Packard servers, telling me to "learn Unix." And I did, as fast as I could possible handle. I think I went home with a headache every single day for six months.

I had always wanted to study Unix. Back in the 80s I knew a fellow who worked at AT&T in the Unix group at the Denver, Colorado facility, and for a little bit I was part of the group of temporary employees. But they had a hard workforce cap (a freeze on hiring of new full-time employees), and I couldn't find a way in. I think, frankly, I gave up too easily. I should have stayed in the temporary worker pool, and created a reputation of being reliable, hard-working, cooperative, and smart. Stuff likes that opens doors to the "who you know" part of the equation. But now, in northern Virginia and ten years later, this was my big chance.

Next thing I knew I had a career in computer security. Who'd have guessed? It was a high time for us geeks too: the dot-com boom was at full throttle, and people were moving jobs and getting a 20 to 30 percent boost (or more) in salaries. Demand for engineers was sky-high.

Most of the team eventually left for other gigs, including my mentor. I went off for a bit to a place out of Gaithersburg, Maryland. Then at my old company, I applied for and was given a promotion to internet administrator on the corporate network team.

This had been a goal of mine, but the previous internet admin had burned a lot of bridges pulling ego-related, manipulative crap on the executives. He also didn't know what he was doing, as I discovered after three months of just trying to figure out what he'd done. I spent that time getting a feel for where things stood before I started revamping, upgrading, cleaning, and configuring the network. This is the sort of dirty work every computer security engineer needs to do: be hands-on, gain some reality on how things actually fit together, and learn how to be quick, efficient, accurate, and in the process avoid interrupting services. But the executives had been burned so badly that the job and role was no longer what it used to be - I had no real say in matters; I had become a keyboard lackey.

Then a friend/former co-worker of mine tried to recruit me for a job at a hot new security company. I wasn't ready at the time, and declined, but a few weeks later my buddy/mentor Scot came a callin', trying to recruit me for a different job at the same company! This time I couldn't refuse.

It was only five years after my new career started when I took the job at NFR Security as VP of Support Services, making nearly eight times what I was when I started. Whoa! Where the hell did that come from? Looking back, I think I was just desperate. I had just hit that point in life where knew I needed to hunker down and make tracks.

It was sort of meant to be. Hell, back in high school, in the late '70s, we had teletypes (basically oversized printers), and I was learned how to program in BASIC, Fortran, and COBOL. My buddies and I would even stay after school writing our own games, some of which became pretty popular with the other students.

At the time (the mid-late 70s) East Coast colleges and universities sucked ass for anything interesting in computers, and I couldn't find one (that would take me) with a computer science degree that focused on anything but dry programming - the kind you do for banks and telephone companies. The place to be for the cool stuff was around Silicon Valley (Berkeley, Stanford) but I didn't know it at the time. Even then, my grades just weren't good enough for those places, and my SAT scores were a disappointment to everyone, including me.

I should say now I had fallen way short of family expectations. I was "supposed to be smart," and I was when I was younger, back when my brain worked right. It was a hell of a thing. Also, that year spent out in Walla Walla put me a year behind, effectively, as they had no advance placement courses whatsoever (in junior high I was already taking AP English and Math), so when I returned, I was a year behind all of my friends, and I think I kind of gave up.

So there I was in New Zealand, twenty-three years later, a total mess again, pedaling along trying to figure things out, what had gone so wrong this time around, and why I felt so damned bad.

The country does things differently, for sure. They've got the Queen of England on their currency, for one. There are five, ten, twenty, fifty and hundred-dollar notes, with everything else in coins: five, ten, twenty and fifty cent pieces, plus one and two-dollar coins. Never saw a penny coin. Taxes are included in all purchases, with everything rounded to the five-cent mark. What you see is what you pay.

The food and prices are kind of crazy as well. Lobster and clams and such are available, of course, but more expensive for the natives than what we pay per pound for lobster up in Maine. Tea and coffee and cakes (meaning, crackers, and even their cookies are really crackers with chocolate chips in them) is a regular thing, and it's normal to stop in the middle of the day to take a break and indulge. Very British.

Lots of different seafoods are listed on the menus, of course. Very good salmon fishing is available, as well as world-class trout fishing expeditions. "Chips" are french fries and food on the average bar menu is very heavy, like poached eggs over fries with two big sausages on the side. I exaggerate only a little, though light meals can be found. Spices are found in lamb curries, though not in much else. Vineyards cropped up everywhere a few decades back, so good wine is fairly common and cheap, as is cheese (first-rate stuff too!).

I spent an extra day in Timaru, recovering. It was fall and the rains were coming, though riding in the rain is a joyful thing compared to the hot sun. I bought a small pack for the top of my front pannier that could easily be detached and carried, with enough room for my camera and lenses as well as snacks and stuff. This way I could take day trips, leaving the heavy bags back in the hotel room. I also picked up dedicated riding shorts and shirt along with a windbreaker.

Chapter Four - Oamaru and Points South

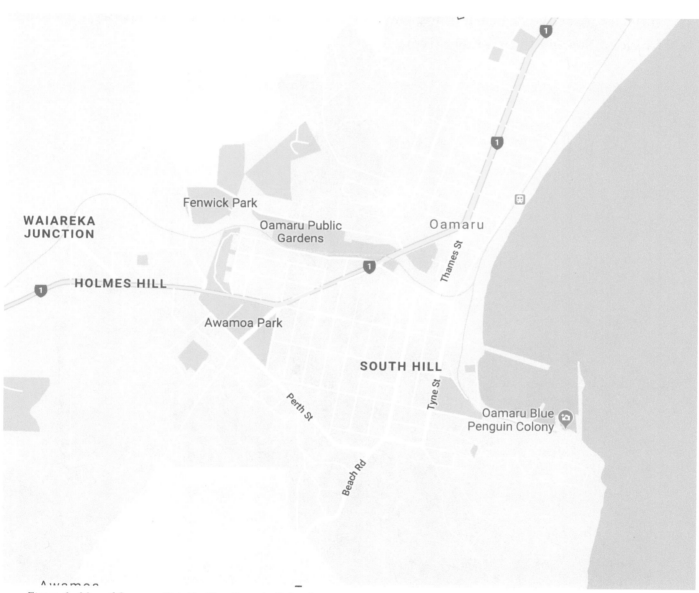

Figure 6 - Map of Oamaru. Note the Blue Penguin Colony!

It was an eighty-eight-kilometer ride to Oamaru. That's over fifty miles, with a bunch of hills to overcome at the outset, but I had a nice wind at my back for the last twenty. I managed to hike my max speed up to twenty-eight kilometers per hour and maintain that for a while. Total time was five and a half hours, so that's an average of sixteen kilometers an hour. Not bad, considering.

It was a beautiful day, with great countryside: rolling hills, yet more sheep (yes, friends, they are kind of cute and fuzzy), lots of cattle, with the Pacific Ocean just to my left. There were fast-moving waters with inlets and side jaunts and foliage, all which divided the mouth of a huge river.

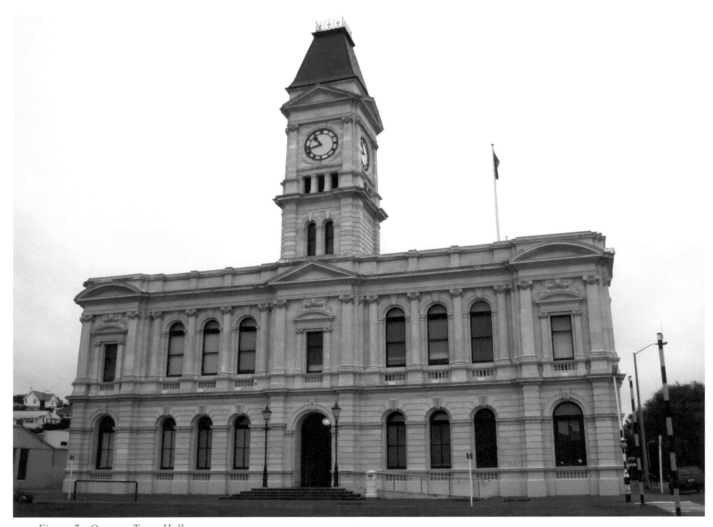

Figure 7 - Oamaru Town Hall

Oamaru has the largest collection of Victorian-style buildings in the country. It is in a small valley surrounded on all sides by a ridge, with many of the houses built up on top allowing them a direct view of the water. It was the most beautiful town I'd seen in the country.

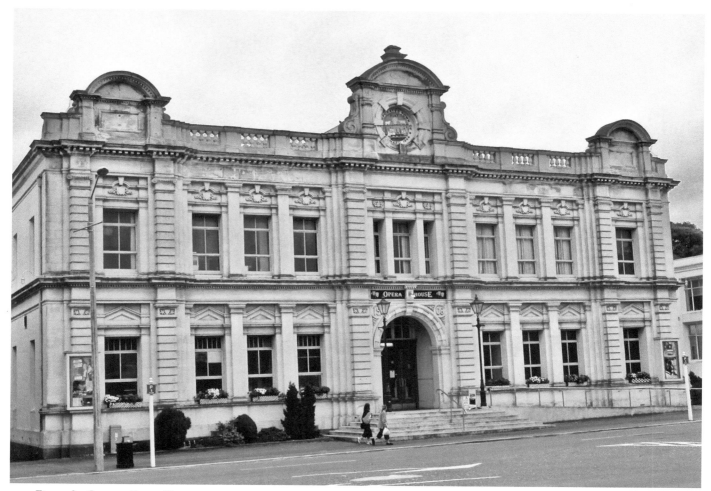

Figure 8 - Oamaru Opera House

I stayed in a backpackers near the center of town. The manager restored vintage bicycles, as in the big-wheeled ones (called *penny-farthings*) and rode them all over the place. He was even the captain of a team of riders. An interesting chap. One advantage of staying in these places is there are frequently common rooms/sitting areas where people gather to talk. I met a fellow from Ireland on vacation, and a girl from Japan there learning English. Apparently New Zealand and Australia are the places to go if you're young and Japanese and want to learn the language.

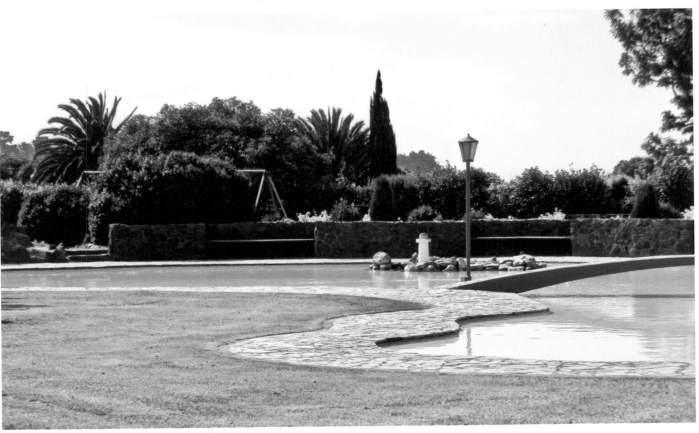

Figure 9 - Oamaru, near the backpackers

I discovered a small museum with some antique cars. Nothing truly special (but then, what do I know?) but fun.

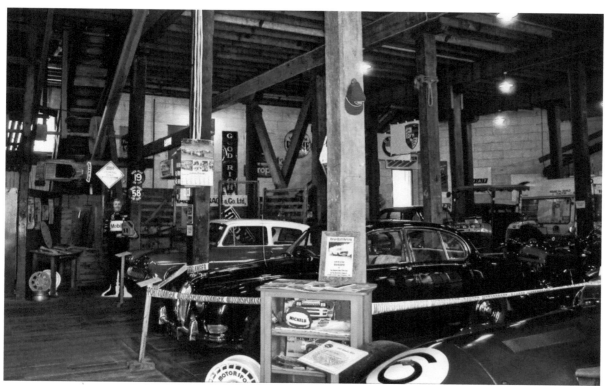

Figure 10 - Oamaru Car Museum

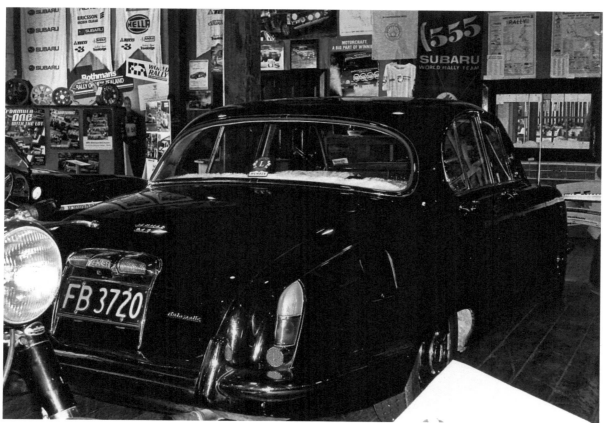

Figure 11 - Old Shaguar

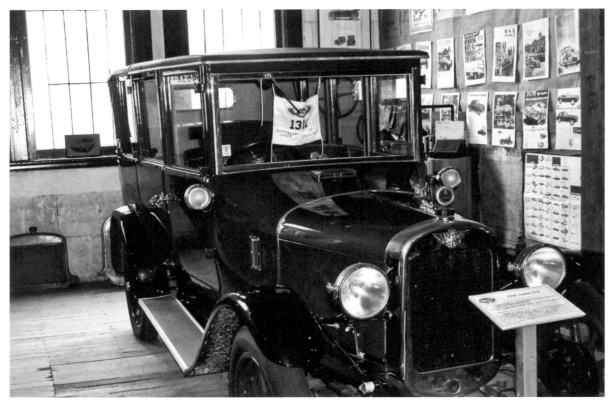

Figure 12 - 1926 Austin 12/4

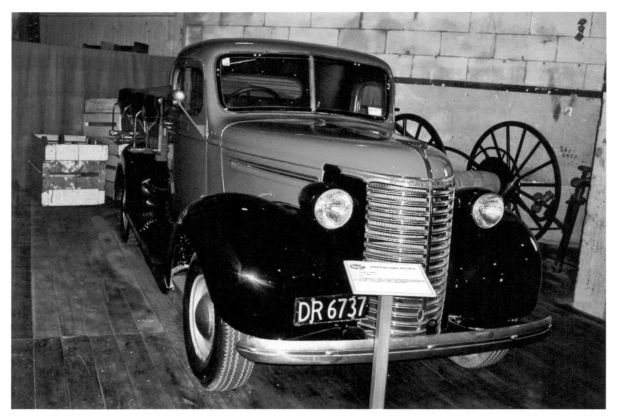

Figure 13 - 1939 Chevy

I spent two nights there, then left Sunday for my next stop, Palmerston, before the final fifty-five-kilometer ride to Dunedin. This was supposed to be easy, but it turned into more like sixty kilometers of rolling hills—not gently rolling hills, but steeply rolling hills, one after another. I found a stop—a place to rest—at Moeraki, where these weird, almost perfectly round boulders are found down on the beach. (Should have taken pictures.)

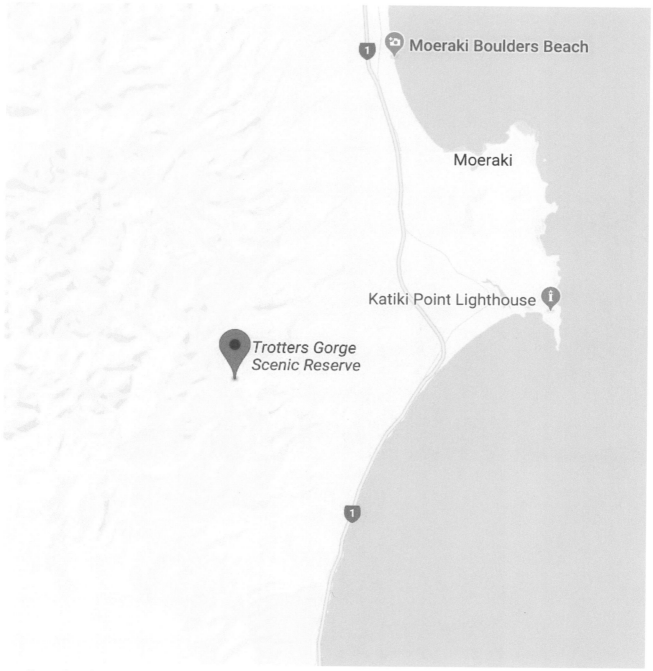

Figure 14 - The Trotter's Gorge "Shortcut"

I made a mistake of taking a shortcut that was not. It seemed that way on the map, and technically, by distance, it was. Trotter's Gorge is very beautiful, but it's a friggin' gorge, which means very deep, and that means one has to get back out. It was so steep that I ended up pushing my bike for the last kilometer. At the top, I was hoping for nice smooth pavement but instead got a steep, winding, twisting gravel road that made for an epic, hair-raising time.

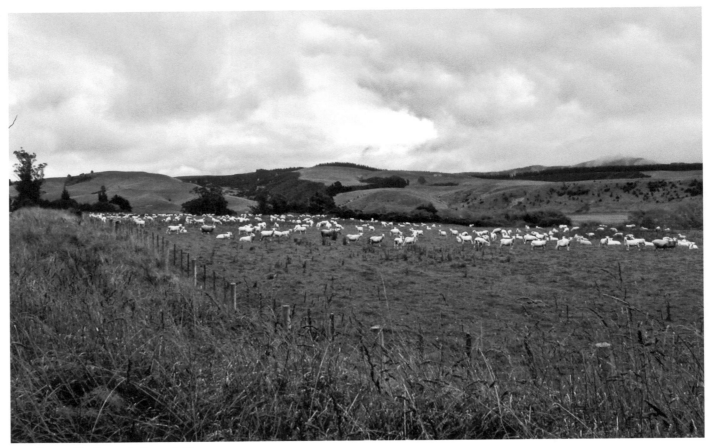

Figure 15 - Towards Trotter's Gorge

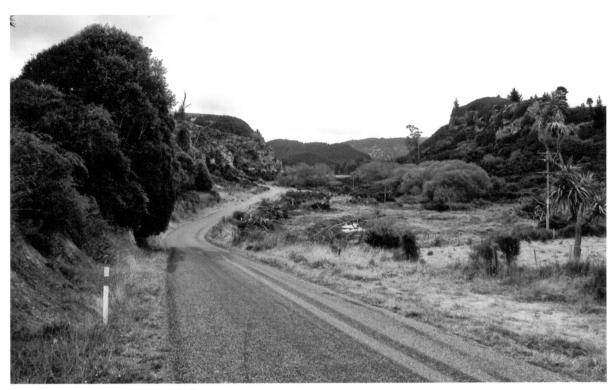

Figure 16 - Road into Trotter's Gorge

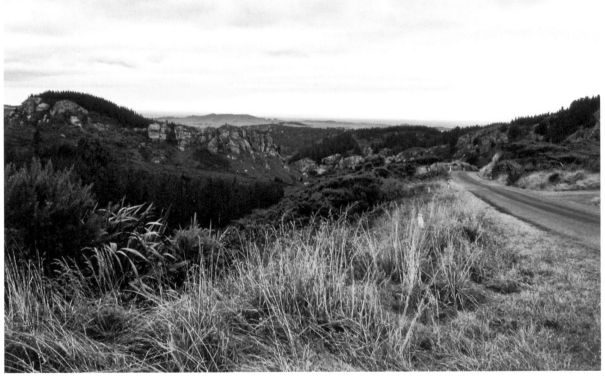

Figure 17 - Trotter's Gorge ahead

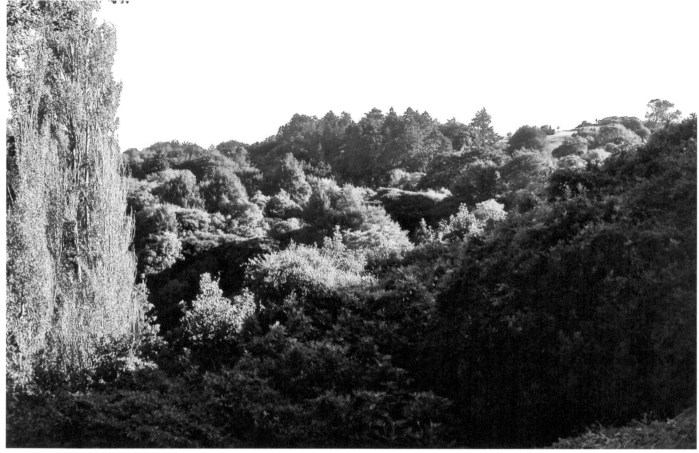

Figure 18 - Deep in the Gorge - Amazing woods

Next up was Palmerston, which sucked. It is a glorified truck stop with a run-down hotel, and everything reeked of smoke. No hot water either. I left promptly in the morning in search of coffee. Then just after the town of Wai-something (turns out it was Waikouaiti), I pushed on to cover more ground with the hope of making my last day to Dunedin that much easier. But then I got a flat tire.

Okay, so no big deal. I carried spare tubes, tools, and of course a pump, so I changed it out and got back on the road. Five hundred meters later I got another flat. Then another, and then I was out of spare tubes!

So I pushed my bike back into town, got some breakfast and coffee, and asked around for a ride into Dunedin to a bike shop. Eventually got one; and this fellow drove like most down there: fast as hell!

It was a good thing I got a ride, as it turned out. That little mountain just north of Dunedin would have made for a 2,100-foot climb. I found out later in my travels that on my rig, even when in better shape, a 1,000-foot climb was more than enough of a workout.

Chapter Five - Dunedin and Otago Peninsula

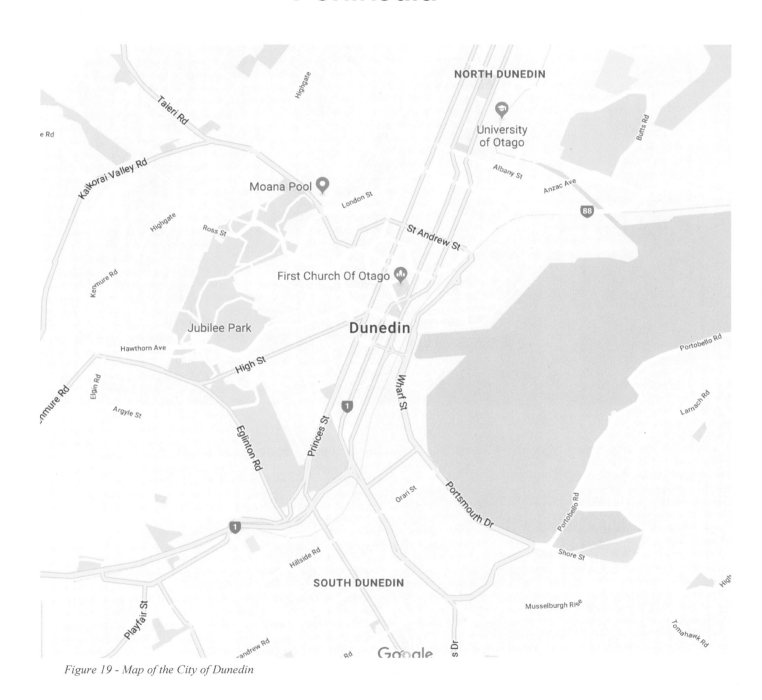

Figure 19 - Map of the City of Dunedin

Dunedin is a city of hills, with the harbor the remains of an old volcano. It also has the world's steepest street.

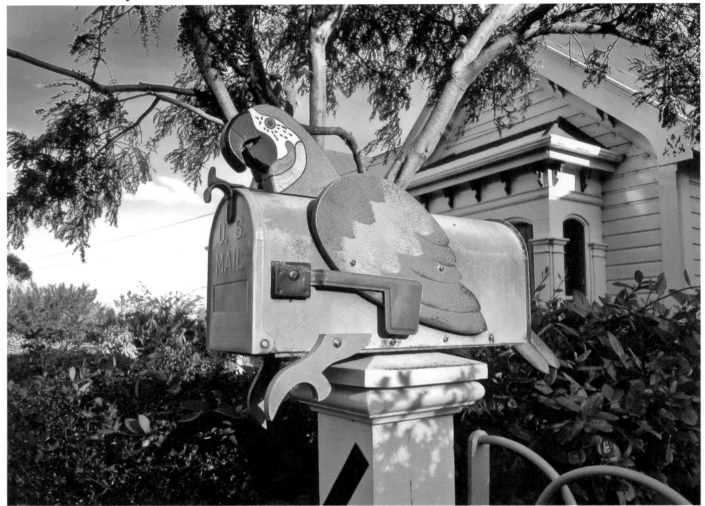

Figure 20 - Dunedin mailbox

I dropped my bike off at a local shop. Turned out there's a strip inside the wheel that covers up the end of the spokes, and while I was careful to put it back right, it was failing to protect the tubes. This allowed a few misaligned spokes to puncture the rubber, thus causing a flat. The strip was replaced with one a bit tougher, the wheels were made round again, and the tube supply was restocked.

I had one other little issue: my right collar bone was killing me, so I found a local massage place right away. The woman there had to use her entire body weight to push it back into place. It's weird when one of your bones goes "click." I had been overcompensating for my weak knee by attempting to take the stress off of it with my shoulder.

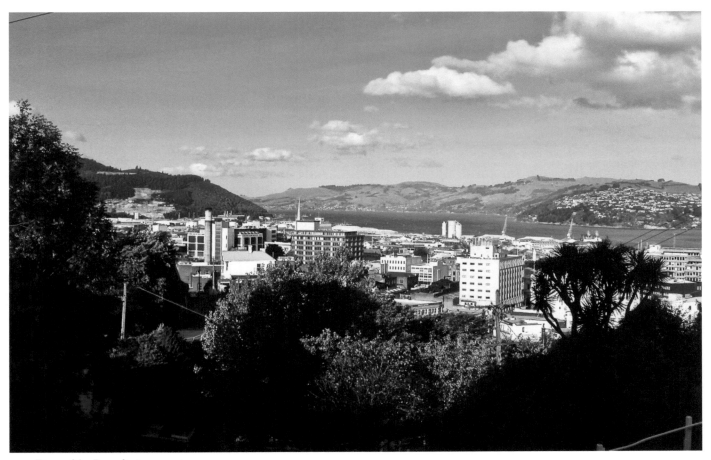

Figure 21 - Dunedin town center

Ah, the knee. Way back in the spring of 1978, when some friends and I were playing soccer, I attempted to do a scissors kick, just trying to copy a buddy, and dislocated my knee. I gave a shout of pain, fell to the ground, then lay there, quite still. Didn't hurt too much, but it didn't help when a klutzy friend, coming over to check me out, accidentally kicked my right foot. DOH!

Someone managed to call 911, and the next thing I knew my dentist was looking down at me. He arrived quickly, as he lived closed by, and had driven his rather new and very sporty-looking Datsun 280Z onto the field.

Oh, that guy had it made. I think he had the best-looking, sexiest aides in the entire area. He was a handsome fellow with a successful practice, so I wasn't surprised he was able to attract plenty of interest from the opposite sex. Anyway, I have fond memories at fourteen of having my teeth worked on by rather buxom women leaning over to get a better look.

While lying in the hospital waiting to get inspected, the kneecap slipped back into place. They put a cast on my leg, and that was that. Since the late '70s, sports medicine has a come way indeed.

Anyway, that was the first time. It went out again in my late twenties, and I needed meniscus surgery then. I thought I had torn an ACL, but fortunately that wasn't the case. Fast forward fifteen years, by the time I was working at the computer security firm, my knee had become unstable again. The right side had become purple and bruised and I could barely walk down the stairs. By the end of this bicycle trip though it was much better, but it would take another fifteen years before the true root cause was found.

I stayed the night in Dunedin at another backpackers that had a dorm-style room for NZ$17. I got the upper bunk, which brought back memories. I hadn't slept in a bunk bed since I was about seven when my older brother and I shared a small room. To this day I still remember falling out of that sucker one night. Uh, OW!

Dunedin is beautiful, and a college town so there's lots of youth and energy. The climate is fairly mild, even at forty-five degrees south of the equator, and while the Pacific is still a bit warm, it can get also quite chilly in the winter, which is probably why the Scots settled here in the first place.

I have a very fond memory of sitting in a coffee house listening to two Kiwi girlfriends chatting in their beautiful, sing-song, somewhat Australian accent (but much nicer to my ears), and not understanding a word they were saying. Of course, one was a beautiful brunette of just my style, which added much to the spell I was under.

.2

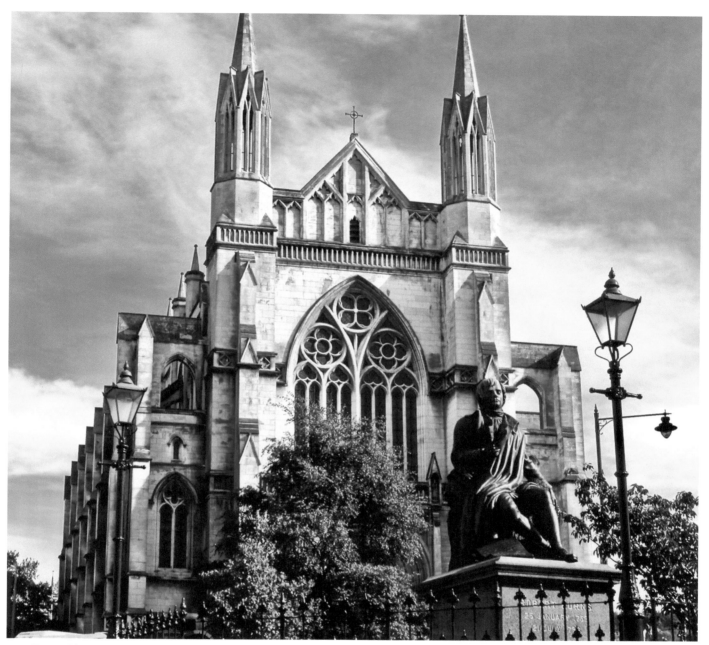

Figure 22 - First Church of Otago with a statue of Robert Burns

Another bit of fun was getting truly hot Hindu food and not being able to finish—I had, after all, asked for "real" hot, not tourist hot. They were happy to deliver and watch me sweat in the process.

Figure 23 - Dunedin Harbor

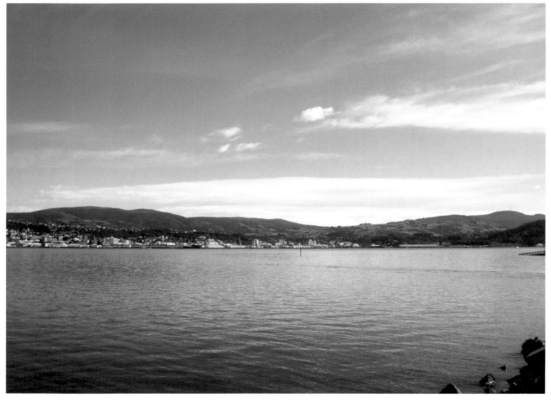

Figure 24 - More of Dunedin Harbor

Dunedin is at the mouth of a long harbor about five miles long and ranging in width from half a mile in close and expanding out to a full mile along the way to the ocean. Defining the south is the Otago Peninsula, which works its way east by northeast. There's a variety of interesting birds about, including albatross. (And if you're now hearing in your head John Cleese from the old *Monty Python* TV shows attempting to sell an "Albatross!" then yer okay with me.)

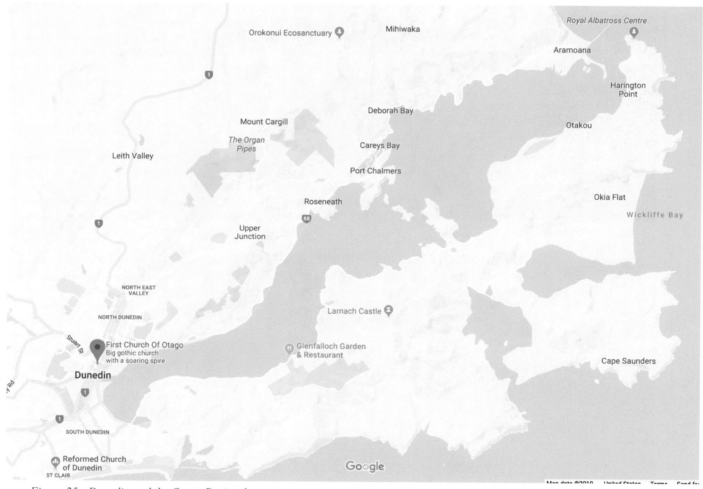

Figure 25 - Dunedin and the Otago Peninsula

I took a "day off" and rode out the peninsula. It's about thirty-five miles long, but flat, so the going was fairly easy, though as you bend around the different harbors the wind can be pretty tough. It's sparsely settled, with mostly sheep and cow farms.

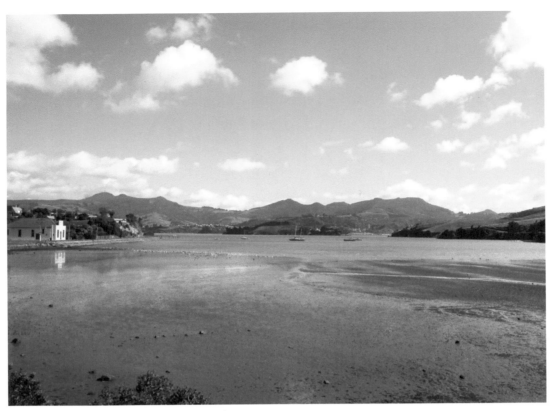

Figure 26 - On my way out the Peninsula

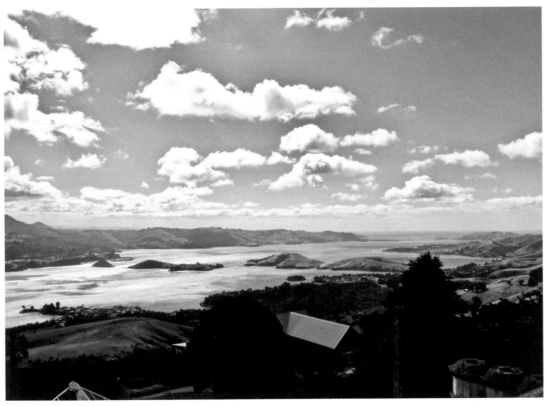

Figure 27 - Otago Peninsula

I did the touristy thing of getting an off-road trip in a local's Land Rover. We traveled around his land which covers roughly seven hundred acres, some of which borders the Pacific and ends in a beautiful lighthouse on a cliff.

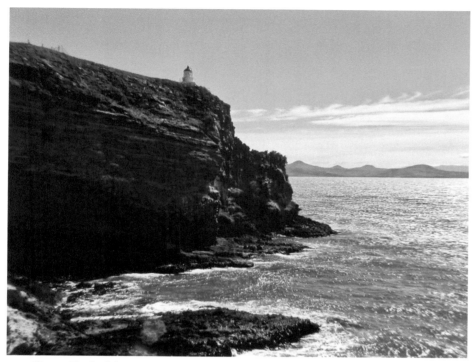

Figure 28 - Lighthouse at tip of Otago Peninsula

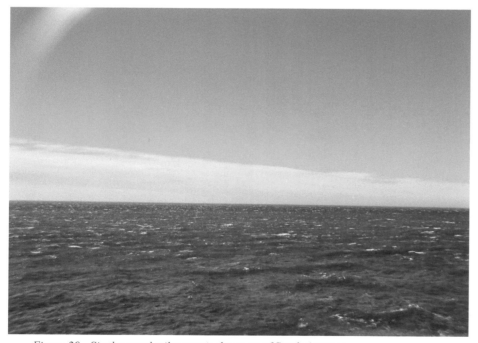

Figure 29 - Six thousand miles east is the coast of South America

I also visited Lornach Castle, which is really a very large house and amazing grounds built on top of one of the ridges that make up the spine of the peninsula. Surrounded by carefully tended gardens and mature trees, at one time in the past it had a very clear, defensive view of the inlet. It was built by a banker who made his money the old-fashioned way: from a gold rush. Yep, gold was discovered in them thar hills, and a narrow-gauged railroad was built up into the hills to ferry workers and ore back and forth. I found out that the train still runs quite a distance in, but thereafter the tracks had been pulled up and turned into a hiking/riding trail. Ooohh, aaaah. Sounded like just my kind of thing.

The ride up to the castle was steep and into a howling wind. The best I could do was to get along about fifty meters before having to stop, gag, and rest before proceeding. I made it about half the three-kilometer distance before my legs gave out, so I walked/pushed my bike the rest of the way.

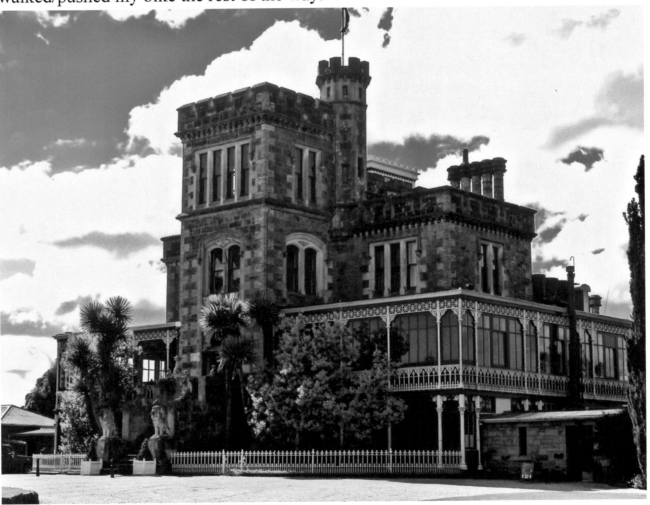

Figure 30 - Lornach Castle

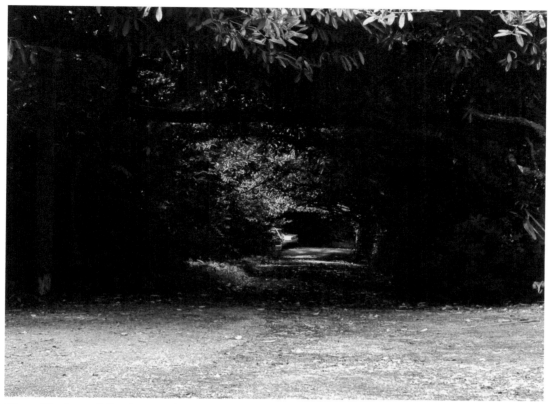

Figure 31 - Lornach Castle grounds

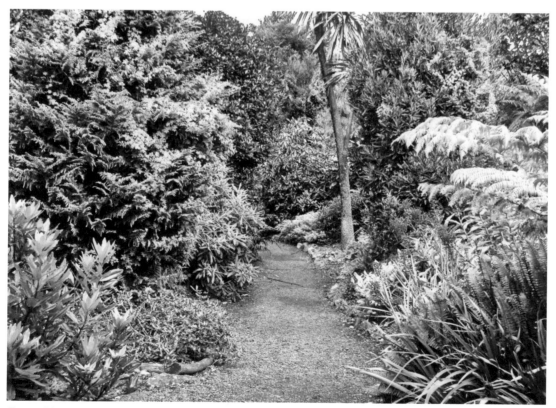

Figure 32 - Amazing gardens

The next day I desperately wanted to see the flocks of albatross that gather out at the end of the peninsula, but my legs were not ready for the fifteen-kilometer ride. Fortunately, a young Swiss couple staying at the backpackers offered to bring me along on their little driving tour, and I happily accepted.

Unfortunately, it turns out one can only see the damn birds by booking a tour in advance. Like, way in advance, and the royal albatross colony was on the other side of a hill and totally out of view. All I saw were a couple floating around way up high, but I did get a good pic of a seal trying to sun himself despite the gaggle of tourists.

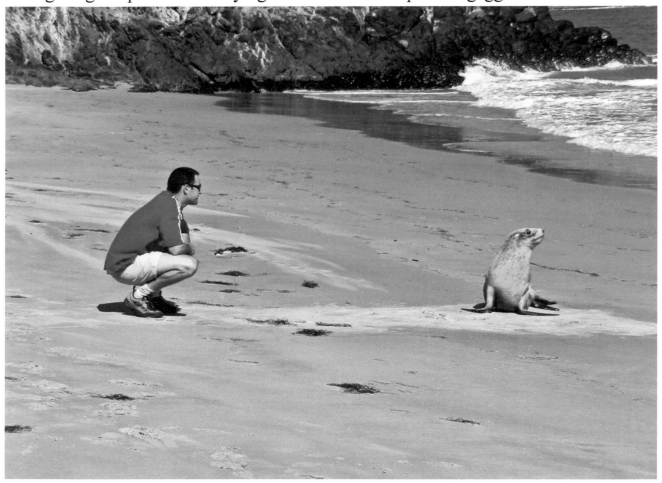

Figure 33 - Dude - you're like, so not mellow.

I went by the local aquarium and got a tour that was hosted by the owner of the backpackers I was staying in. (Nice little coincidence there - but it does seem like everyone knows everyone.) Saw some eels, rays, crayfish, muscles, clams, sea horses, and other cool fishies. But I wanted to make Wanaka by Easter weekend for the South Pacific Warplanes Air Show (a very big event), so I didn't tarry longer.

Chapter Six - The Rail Trail

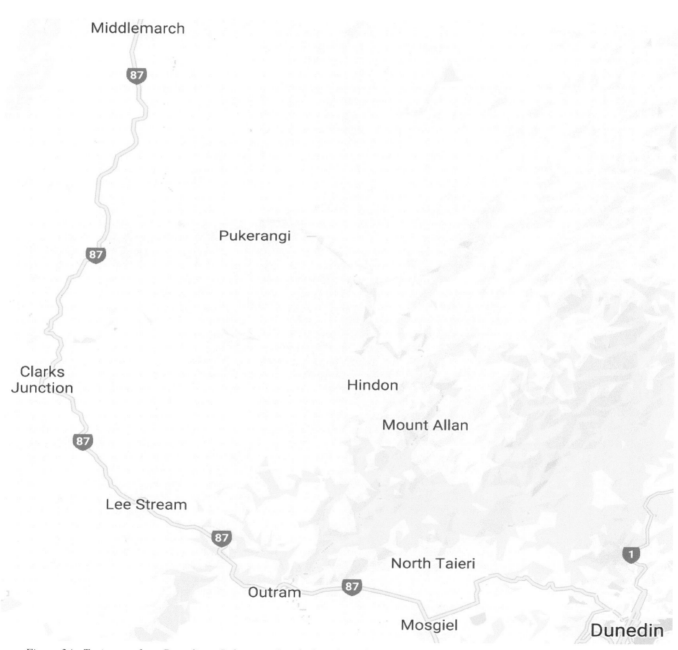

Figure 34 - Train runs from Dunedin to Pukerangi; I picked up the rail trail at Middlemarch

The old gold rush train only goes one hundred kilometers now, along a narrow, twisting gorge. The locomotive was completely refurbished, and huffed and puffed happily up the grades, towing passenger cars that were beautifully made.

I met a couple at the station that were sailing around the world by themselves, struck up a brief conversation, and expressed my admiration and envy. They seemed a little offish, so I left them alone. Later I found myself seated right across from them, and we ended up getting along famously, as the Kiwis say. They even invited me for a sail assuming I ever got back up the Auckland way. Sadly, I lost their information and never was able to take them up on this offer. Big sigh.

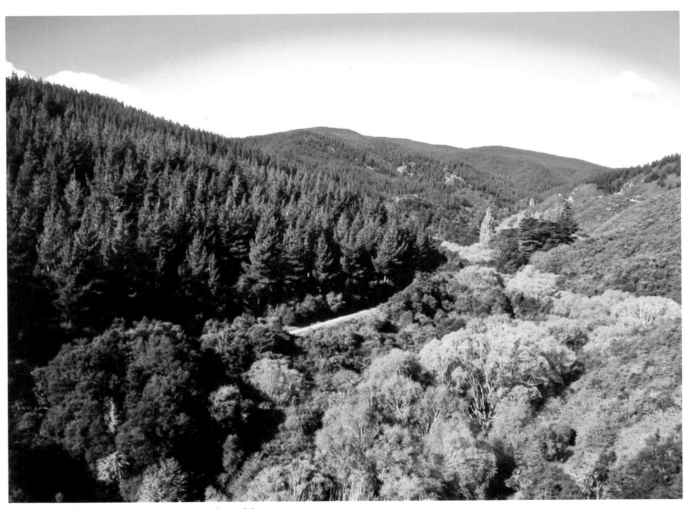

Figure 35 - Looking west out the window of the train

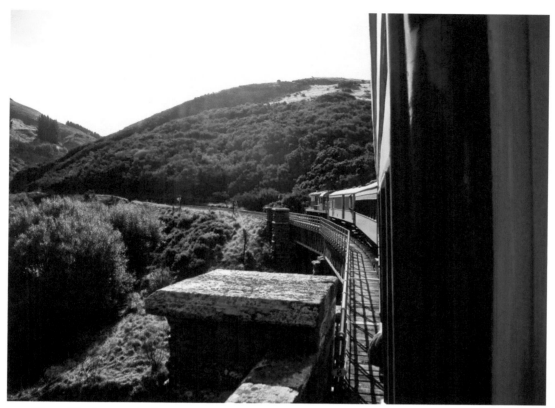

Figure 36 - Across a bridge

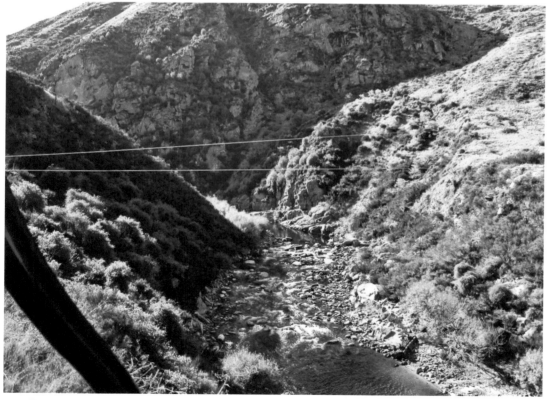

Figure 37 - Looks ripe for gold panning

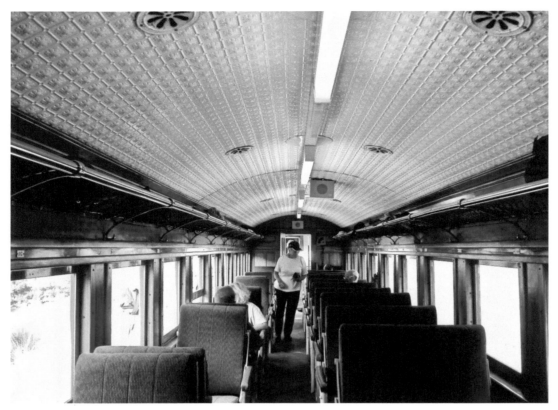

Figure 38 - Beautiful old rail car

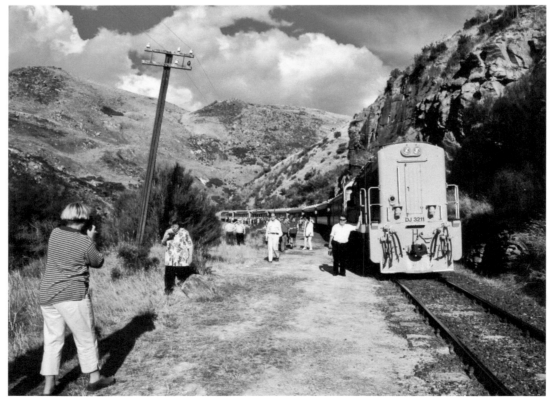

Figure 39 - End of the tracks

The journey ended at the little town of Pukerangi, at which we all disembarked. The rest of the track had long since been pulled up and sold as scrap metal, so now people use the remaining 150-kilometer distance of crushed gravel path for biking, running, walking, horseback riding, etc. It crosses quite a bit of ranch and farm land, and more than a few cow gates, forcing one to dismount to get through.

Coming off the train my legs were still pissed at me, but there was a lot of riding yet to do, first along some roads to the trailhead, then to make Middlemarch for the night in another backpackers. It was the last non-windy day for the next three.

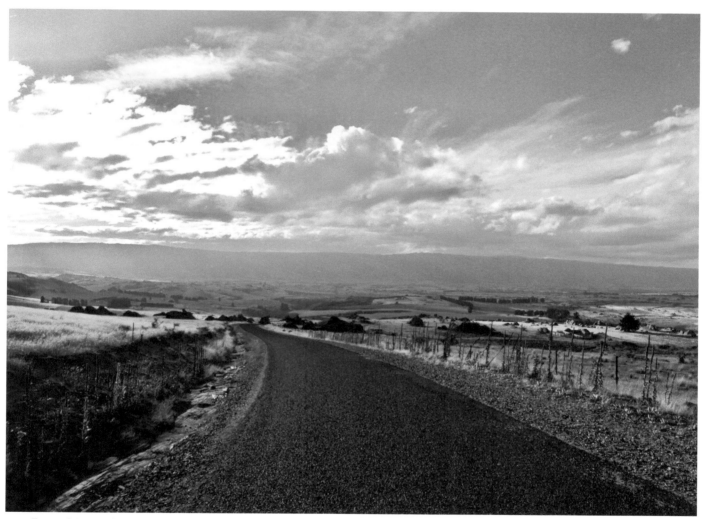

Figure 34 - Road towards Middlemarch

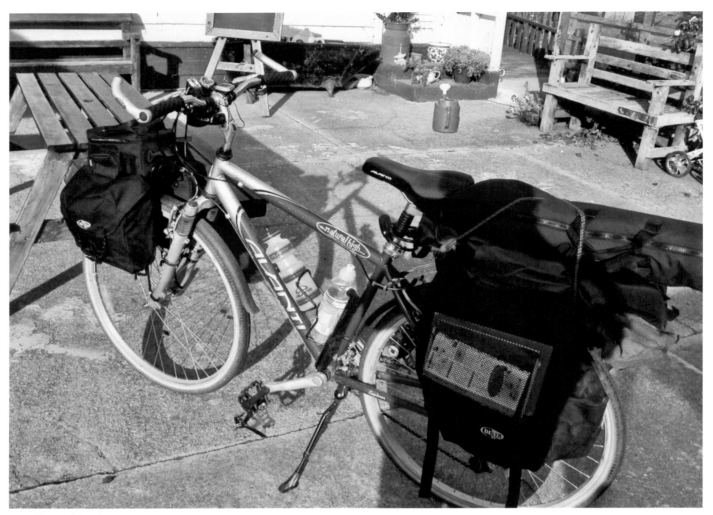

Figure 36 - The rig

My rig, above, is an Avanti, out of Auckland. The purple thing is the case for my little guitar, with the green backpack below it for hikes and such. The front top bag removes easily for day trips or whatever, and also is reachable over the handlebars for a quick snack. The handlebar extensions are climbing bars, which were invaluable. I don't ride with clips or special shoes; yeah, they're more efficient in terms of putting down the power, but I've always felt like my ankle had a good chance of twisting if I fell off.

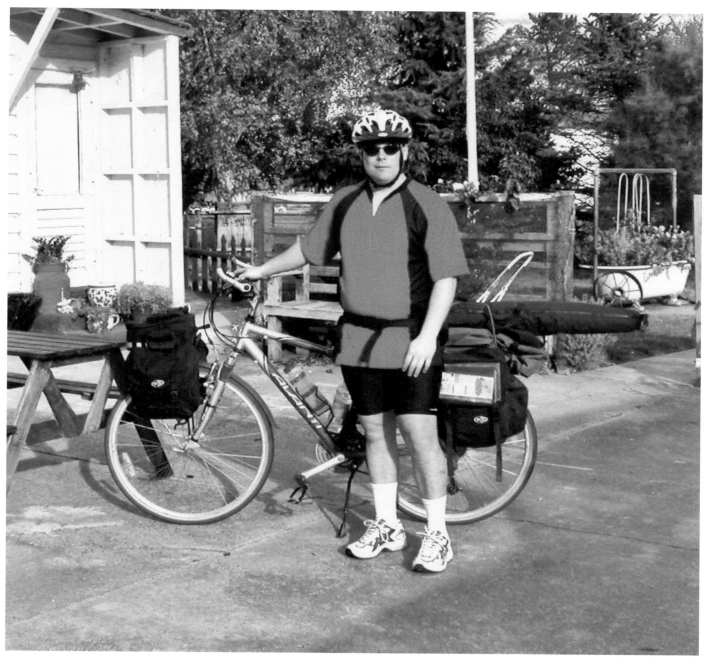

Figure 37 - All geeked out in riding gear

The next day I rode for Pete's Farm Hostel in Waipiata. The terrain reminded me a lot of southeastern Wyoming and northeastern Colorado: flat, sometimes boring and dry, but open, with big, beautiful skies, and I heard the fly-fishing is world-famous. The rail trail works its way up toward the towns of Alexandria and Cromwell, old gold rush towns as were Queenstown and Wanaka.

51

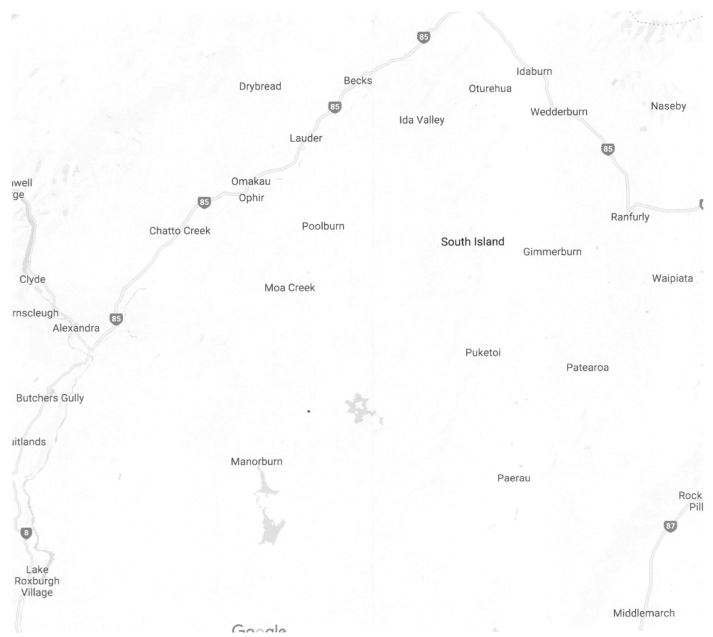

Figure 40 - From Middlemarch to Clyde

I hit a strong wind, first catching me from the west, but as I was going north by northwest, it wasn't too bad, but then it switched around to the north and started increasing in intensity. The last ten kilometers were brutal. I struggled to keep going even in first gear, despite keeping my head down as low as possible. I covered fifty-two kilometers that day. Ugh. By the time I reached my destination, I was completely spent and was barely able to stand. I took the next day off, needless to say.

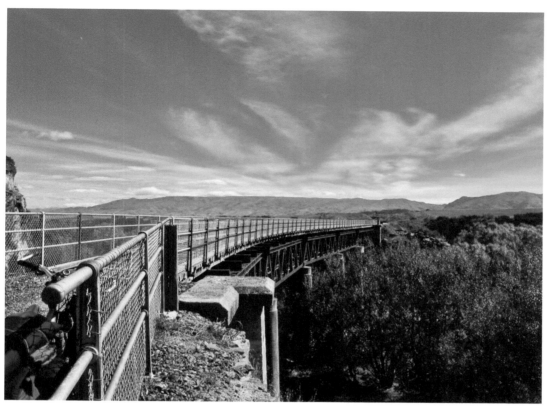

Figure 35 - Beautiful bridge, part of the trail

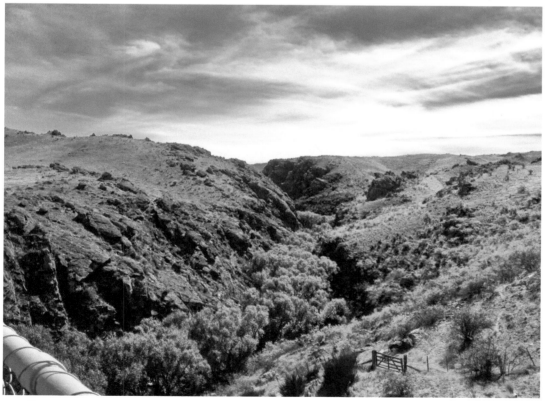

Figure 41 - Pretty ranching country

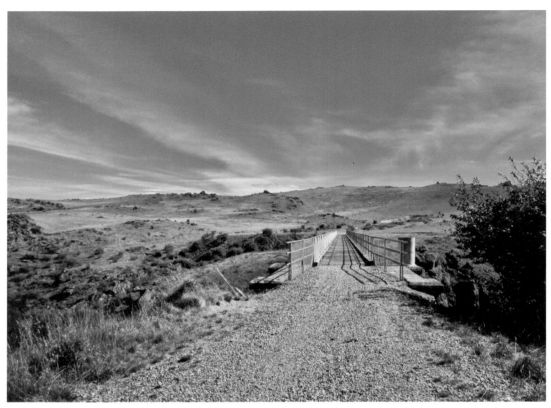

Figure 42 - There's gold in them thar hills!

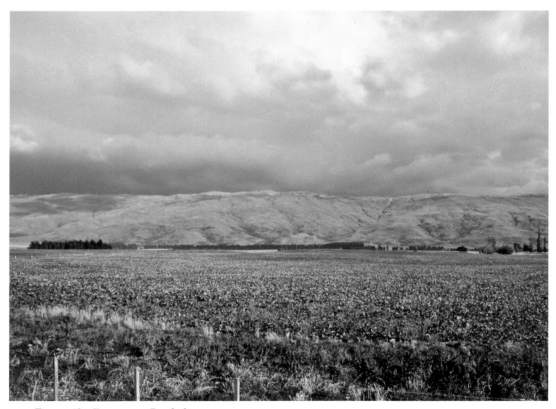

Figure 43 - Farms past Ranfurly

Pete was in a bad mood, as it turned out—a bus full of tourists, who had also requested some food supplies, had canceled, and his food was going to spoil. I cheered him and his helper up with a bottle of wine and some guitar playing and singing. His helper was an Italian woman living in Germany but touring New Zealand trying to find work as a magician—I kid you not!

As for the guitar, mine was from Go-Guitars (go-guitars.com) in California, who are still making fine little instruments that sound good. Mine was a Grande with walnut and a mahogany neck, that when plugged in had a surprising amount of bass. I had been playing for years in coffee shops and open mics, and I'm not half bad, though I never wanted the life (staying up late, playing in smoky bars, traveling all of the time, no real relationships…).

Waipiata, Pete said, was a dead town: there was no good water anymore, so no new houses could be built. But the tourism was excellent, and the local men could charge NZ$500 a day as a fly-fishing guide.

I met a French couple that was traveling by bike and camping their way through New Zealand and Australia. Neat people. The fellow was very relieved when I told him there were entire conversations in Kiwi of which I didn't understand a word. He just though his English was bad!

My next ride was for Ranfurly, a little hub of the area, only eight kilometers away, and I reached it easily as there was little wind. Unfortunately, it kicked up after that, and I had it in my face again until the trail turned west then southwest, but then it started heading a bit downhill. For about fifteen minutes I was in a state of total bliss, going about twenty-four kilometers per hour, flying along with the trail with the wind at my back. After a water break, the wind switched around without letting up, and I struggled on to the next town, Lauder. Again, a fifty kilometer plus day. Crazy.

The next day I left early, just wanting to get to the next big town, in this case Alexandra, only thirty-six kilometers away, to then give my body a break. Fortunately, the wind had died, the weather was warm, and the scenery improved to a mix of gorges and volcanic-looking outcroppings. I actually made it past Alexandra to the next town.

Clyde is yet another ex-gold mining town, located at the base of a dam. Should the dam break, well, there would go Clyde. It is perfect wine country! There was also great food, with one place in the old district having etouffee. Yum! Yes, that's good old Louisiana etouffee in a blues bar/restaurant in the middle of the South Island of New Zealand.

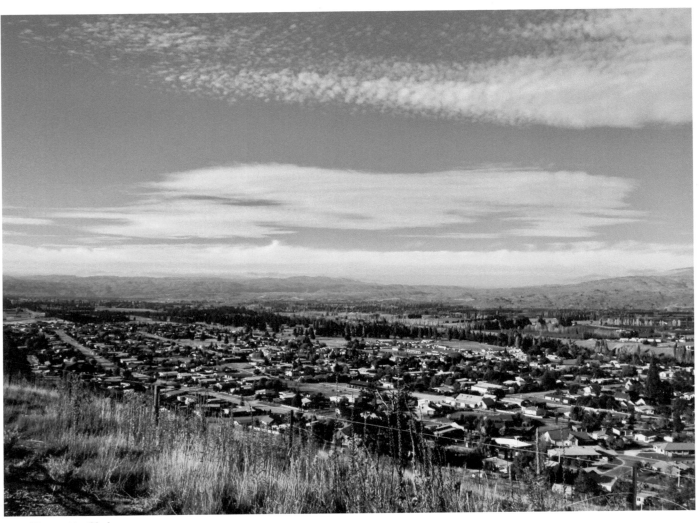

Figure 44 - Clyde

After another break, I made for the next town, Cromwell, which was twenty-five kilometers away. I made it but started getting flats again. The long, hard ride on the rail trail had thrown my wheels out of round, and I ended up having to get a ride to my next destination, Queenstown.

Chapter Seven - Queenstown and Wanaka

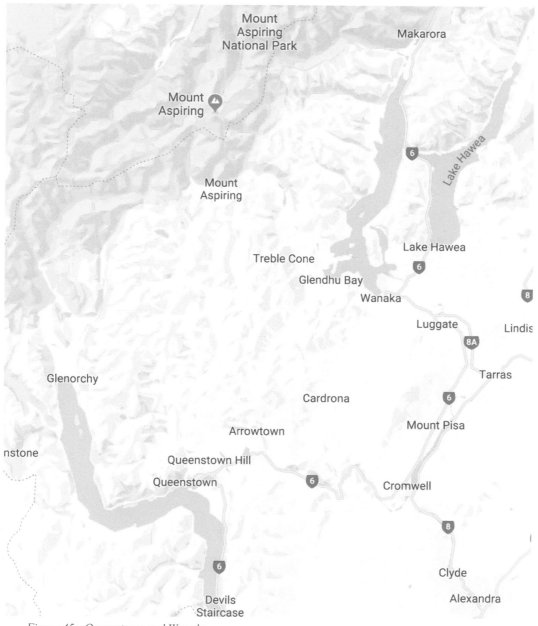

Figure 45 - Queenstown and Wanaka

There wasn't any lodging within one hundred kilometers of Wanaka, where the air show was soon to be held, but I did get a room in Queenstown at a backpackers named Scallywag's. A young Jewish couple I talked to during my travels had stayed there and said it was quite good, so what the hell. It was owned by one of the original base jumpers, and he had pictures of himself in various funny poses, hanging from bottom of the line, having reached its extent.

Yes, extreme sports were born here in Queenstown, the self-proclaimed "Adventure Capital of the World." They've got all kinds of stuff for adrenalin junkies: helicopter skiing and hiking in remote areas, skydiving, jet-boat river trips, you name it. It is located in the southern-middle part of the mountainous, volcanic spine that runs along the western part of the South Island, with peaks that rise up to over twelve thousand feet. They call the area to the north of Queenstown the "Southern Alps" for a reason. I took a longer rest here, played tourist for a while, picking up in their very nice downtown market a beautiful black-and-red 100 percent wool jacket that I still love to this day.

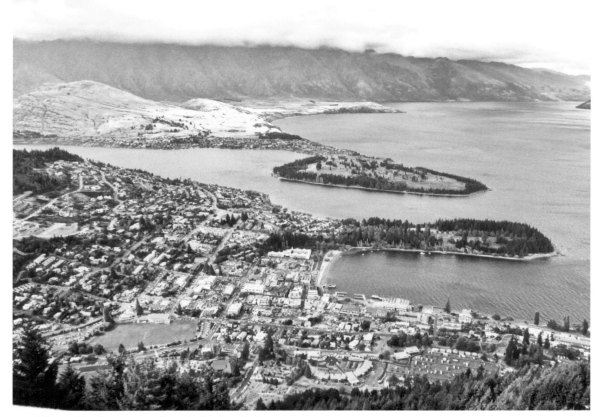

Figure 46 - Queenstown from the backpacker's

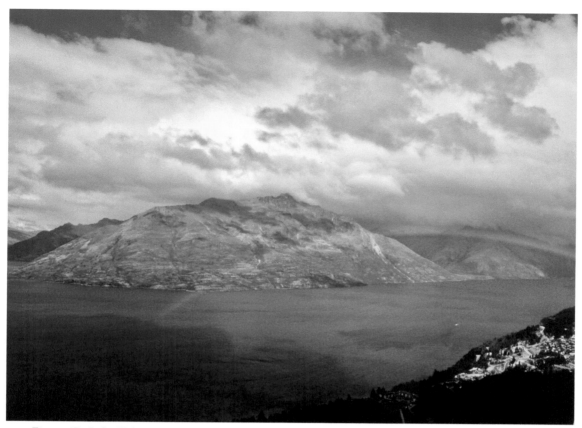

Figure 47 - Lake Wakatipu

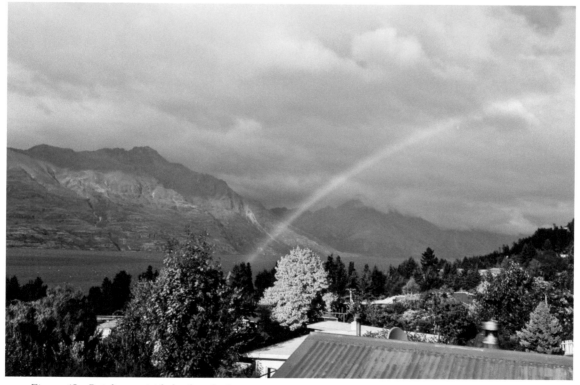

Figure 48 - Rainbow outside backpacker's

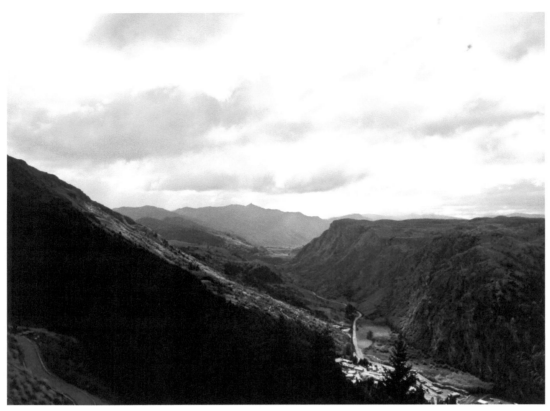

Figure 49 - Looking West

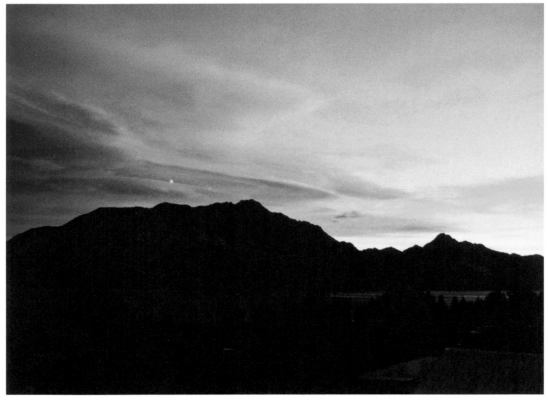

Figure 50 - Sunset over Queensland

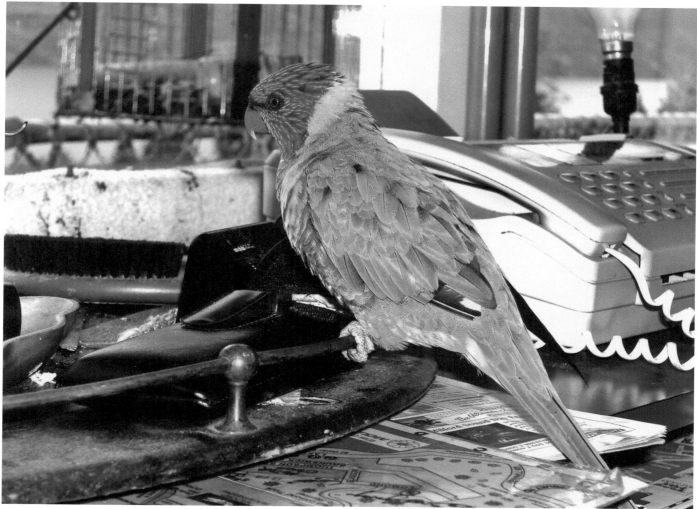

Figure 51 - The house parakeet - friendly bugger!

To the south are towns such as Te Anau, which is the gateway to Fjordland (a series of fjords, totally unpopulated and wild), and then Invercargill on the southern tip, a pretty decent-sized town (around fifty thousand), pretty much the anchor to the region. There are two huge parks to the east of that city. Finally, there's Stewart Island (a.k.a. Rakiura), alone by itself about fifteen kilometers south of the mainland. I never did get down there; it was mid-late fall now (though early April my time), starting to get cold, and I wanted to finish up my ride by about mid-May.

The South Island has no active volcanos. The fault on which New Zealand lies appears to be moving in a north-east direction, breaking apart as it goes. There was a big eruption several years before my trip in the active section of the middle of the North Island, with another occurring in 2012, but I never made it that plateau. From what I've heard, it's worth the trip.

I stayed through Easter then took a bus over to Wanaka for the air show. It's not really that far, but there is a very big climb along the direct route, and the "easy" way was two days out of my schedule. From Wanaka I intended to head over Hast Pass, out of the rain shadow of the Southern Alps, and into the rain forest, i.e., the West Coast. I figured to make it as far as Greymouth before catching a bus up to Nelson, which is at the north end of the South Island. This would leave me a good month to explore the North Island, which was looking really cool: hot springs, geysers, a live little volcano off the shore, more of the indigenous Maori culture as well.

The Wanaka Air Show is biennial, the largest in the southeastern part of the globe. There were a ton of warbirds, almost none of which I recognized. It was a coldish, windy day, with clouds racing over the face of the sun. (I had to edit quite a few of my photos to brighten them up enough to bring out the details.) Toward the end I got very lucky with the picture of the child on his father's shoulder and the P-51 Mustang flying behind. It looks like a toy model in the photo, but that's a live bird there! The very last picture in the series is of the Wanaka Lake and dock area, where I jumped a bus going to the West Coast.

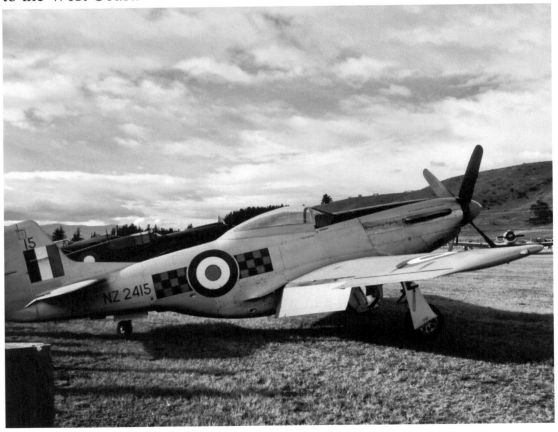

Figure 52 - North American P-51D Mustang

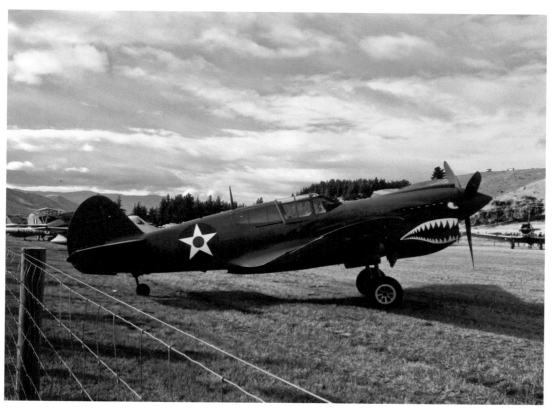

Figure 53 - Vought F4U Corsair

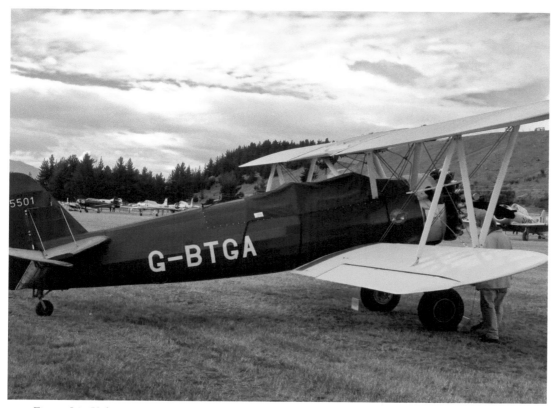

Figure 54 - Unknown

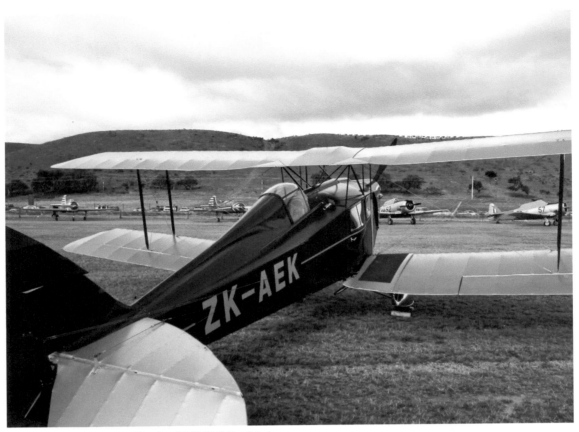

Figure 55 - 1932 De Haviland DH-83C Fox Moth

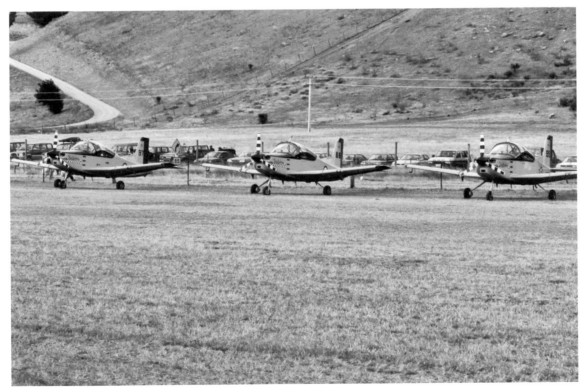

Figure 56 - Stunt fliers

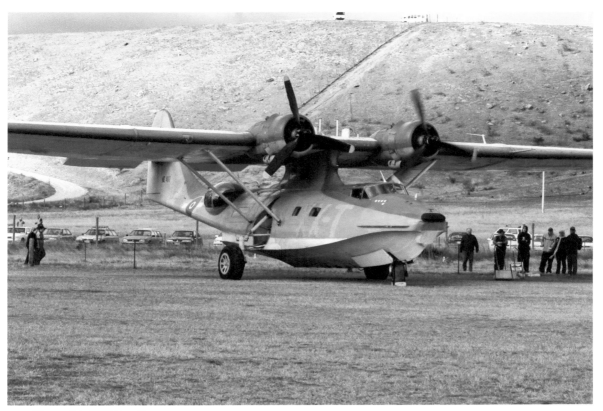

Figure 57 - PBY Catalina

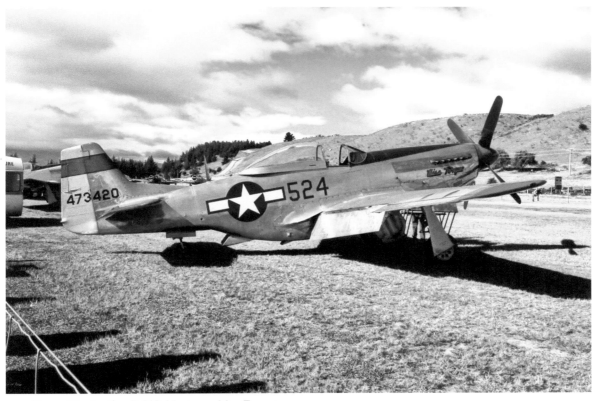

Figure 58 - Another P-51D Mustang - Miss Torque

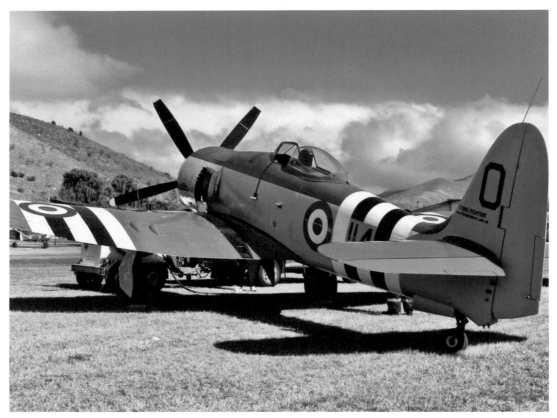

Figure 59 - Another view of a P-51D Mustang

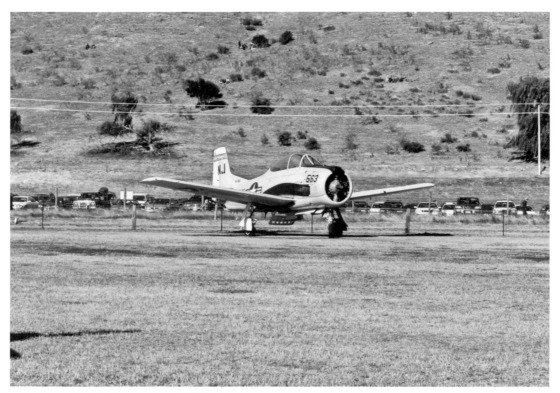

Figure 60 - North American T-28 Trojan

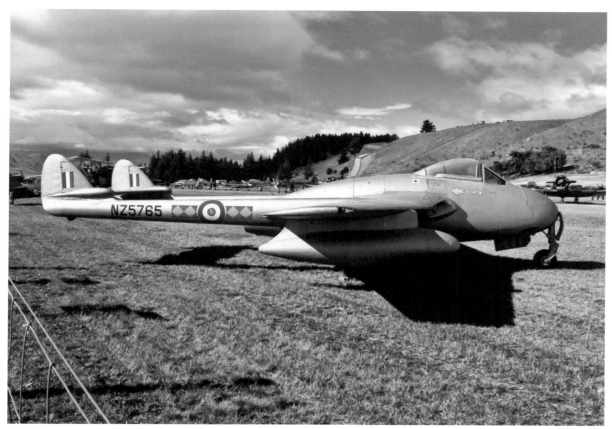

Figure 61 - De Haviland DH100 Vampire

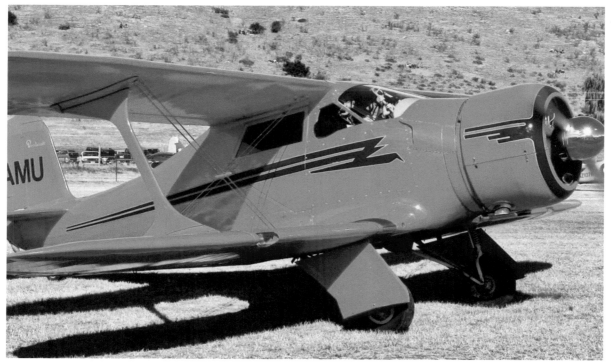

Figure 62 - Modern biplane - looks stable and strong.

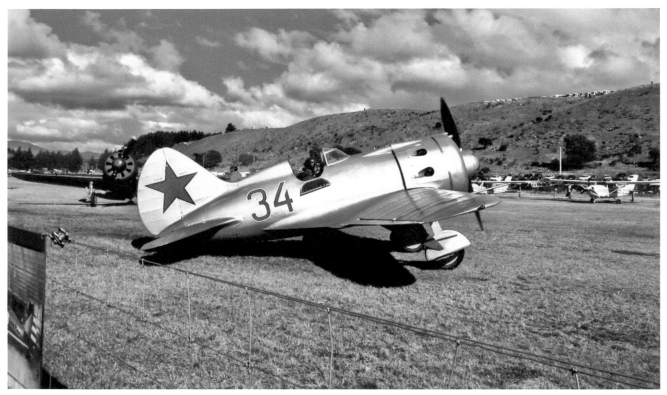

Figure 63 - Polikarpov I-16 ?

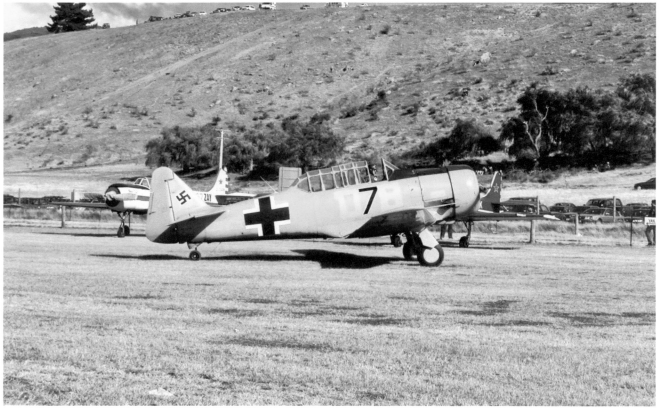

Figure 64 - Fokker D

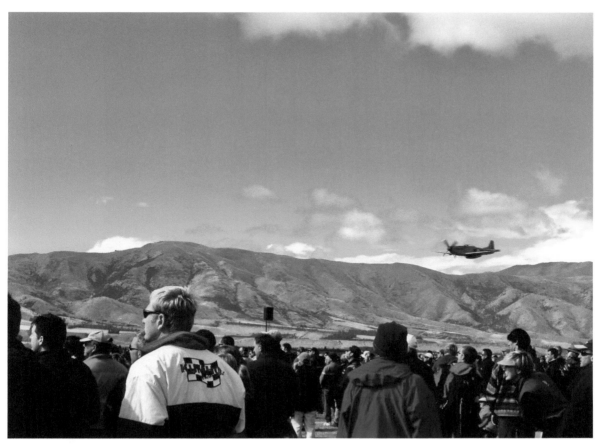

Figure 65 - P-51D Mustang in flight

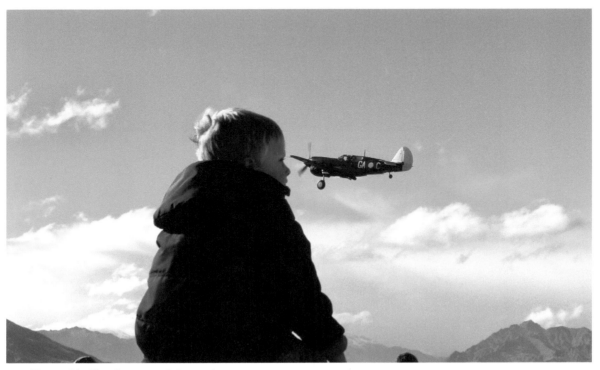

Figure 66 - The plane is real, I swear!

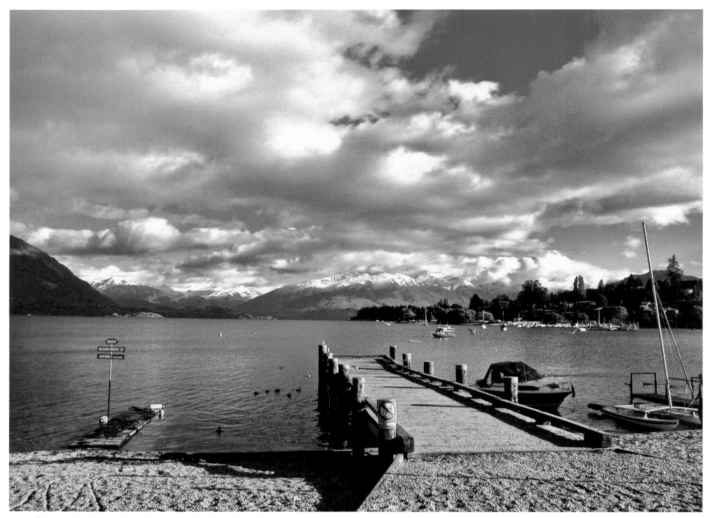

Figure 67 - Wharf leading out into Wanaka Lake

Chapter Eight - The West Coast and Nelson

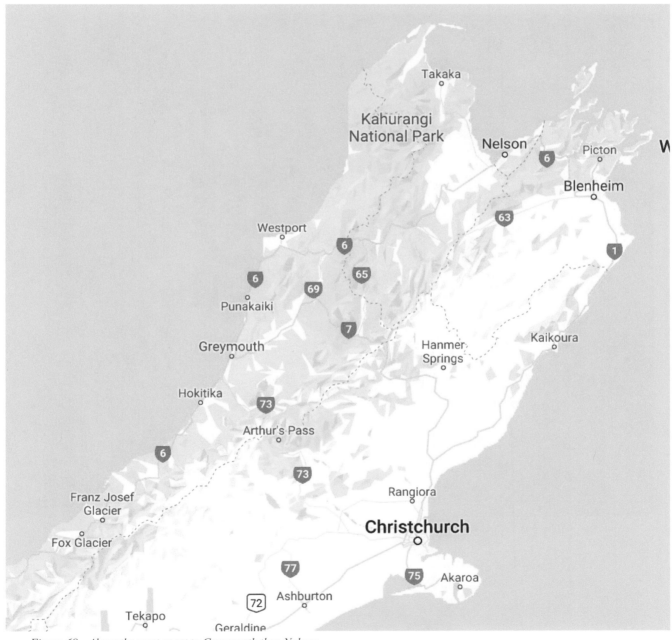

Figure 68 - Along the west coast to Greymouth then Nelson

The next pictures were taken during a bus stop on the way over to the West Coast. Note the sudden, drastic change in scenery! We went up and over a very steep, winding pass, one which I'm very glad I didn't attempt as I watched the driver almost run a fellow bicycler off the road, who was struggling mightily with a heavy rig. Buses are terrible for cyclists: their smooth sides create a strong vortex as they blast by you, making it an effort to even stay upright. And of course like most roads and routes through New Zealand, there was no shoulder, and therefore, no escape.

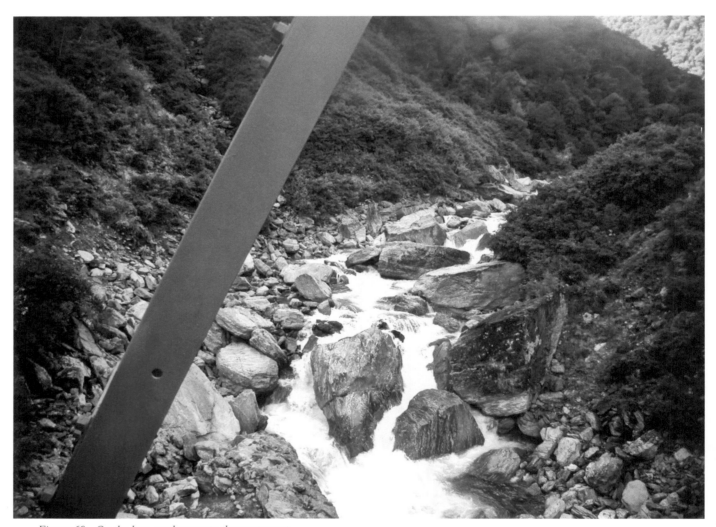

Figure 69 - On the bus, on the way to the west coast

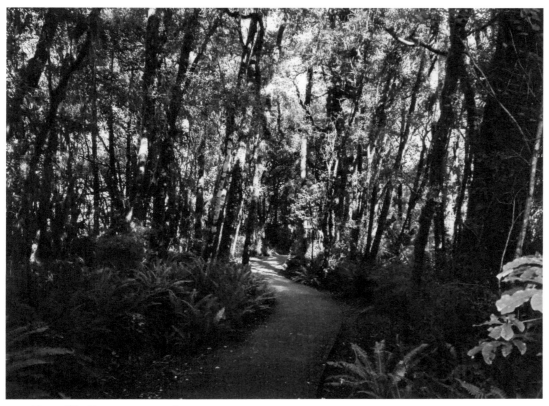

Figure 70 - Rest stop at a park

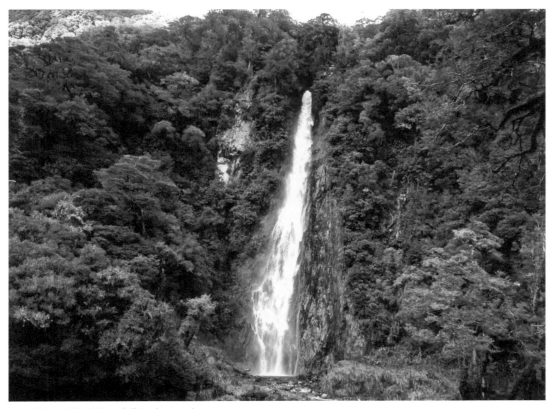

Figure 71 - Waterfall in the jungle.

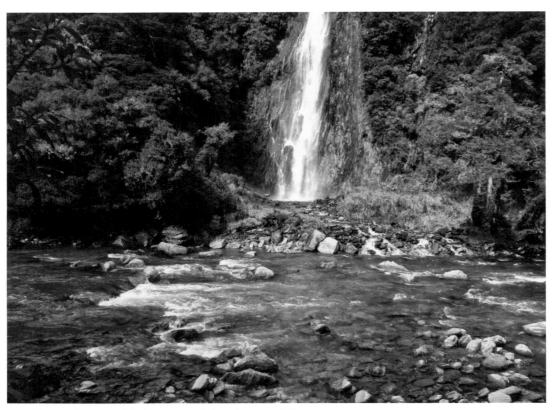

Figure 72 - Beautiful clear stream below the waterfall

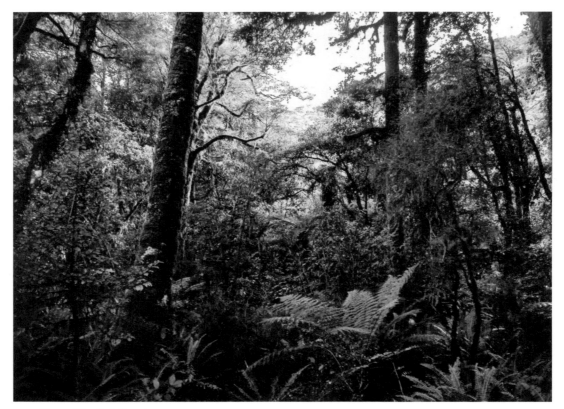

Figure 73 - Rainforest now

On the bus now I had a little time to reflect. I was still quite angry about all of the problems with my last job. What a mess. Egos should never interfere with cooperation, and software design shops like ours require constant communication and lock-step coordination between engineering, quality assurance, marketing, sales, support, and the executive staff. New features should be decided on months in advance; no last-minute "oh we should do this too" crap, and new software releases should be a coordinated effort. Bugs should be tracked, and the big ones fixed before rollout. None of that was going on. It was like herding cats, which meant that people like me and a number of others were working very, very inefficiently, with long hours to boot, attempting to make up for lost ground. What a mess.

Okay, so I'm ranting, even now, seventeen years after the fact. I learned a lot, though, but I had lingering questions about my own performance. Why couldn't I handle the workload? Seemed like I went from healthy to barely functioning in no time. Others seemed to handle the stress much better.

I was mad at the CEO; but it turned out I should have been mad at the founder, who was screwing with stuff constantly and had driven off excellent engineers—the real brains behind the software engine—prior even to my arrival. The CTO was an "idea guy" with a huge ego, and I'm telling you now: idea guys are a dime a dozen. That's not what defines success. Anybody can criticize anything, it takes real guts to make a decision, stick with it, and work stupid hard in a spirit of cooperation with your brethren. There are always plenty of good ideas running around, from all kinds of sources. What makes a company win business is providing the customer what they want, on time, with the features they're looking for and the major bugs figured out.

It also takes humility, gratitude, and the willingness to admit screwups. Well, I'm far from perfect, for sure, and I made my share of bad decisions: I let one of my lead quality assurance engineers bring in a friend from a competing company and allowed that fellow to log onto the network. Doh! This was the excuse people were looking for to finally get rid of me. That's fine; they did me a favor, as it took me another two years before I even started to feel somewhat healthy again.

The West Coast is normally very, very wet and very, very windy, but this year had been quite cool and pretty dry up to this point. Sure enough, we hit Greymouth on the way up the coast and the cold weather hit: forty-five degrees and windy, which is downright freezing when you're used to seventy-five to eighty.

It's a sparsely populated area. Most of it is empty and wild for hundreds of miles. All of the good fishing is off the East Coast, and as it's drier, it's also more livable. If you want to climb a glacier, though, this is where you want to be.

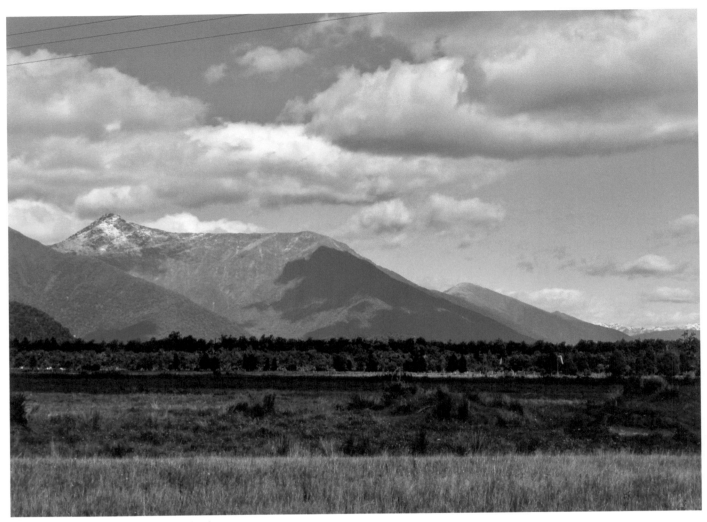

Figure 74 - West coast, looking back east

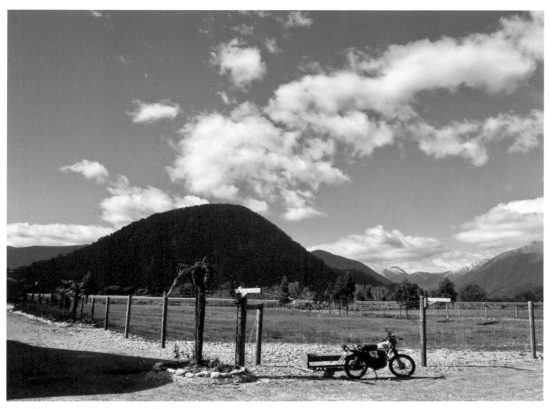

Figure 75 - Near Haast, I believe

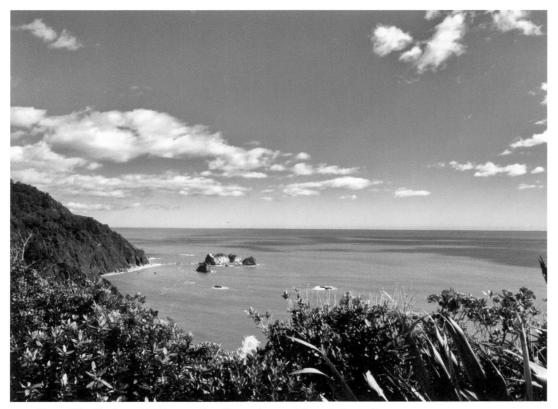

Figure 76 - The beautiful Tasman Sea. Somewhere out there is Australia

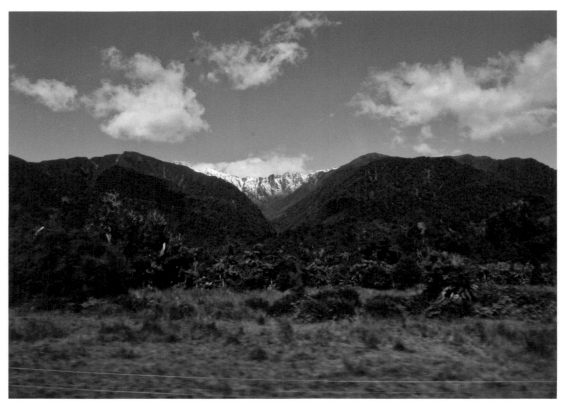

Figure 77 - Some glaciers live way up there

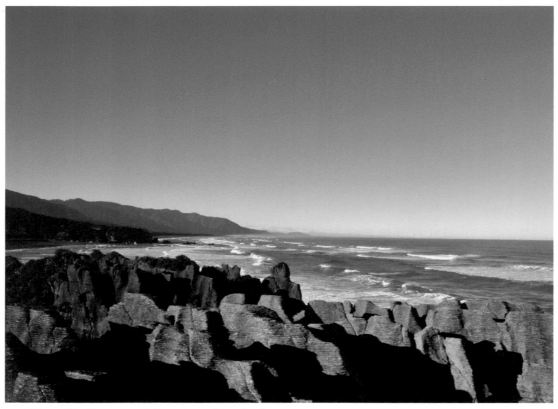

Figure 78 - Strange rock formations along the shore

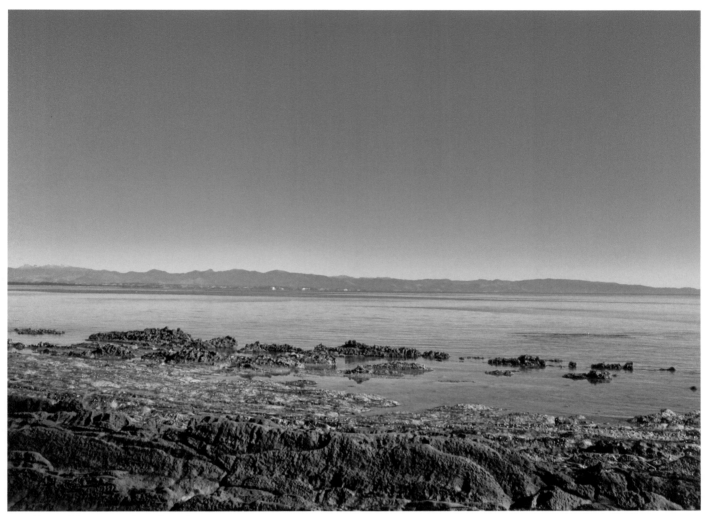

Figure 79 - A pretty bay along the west coast

We reached Nelson the next day. It's considered the gateway to the South Island, a touristy area where one can rent just about anything, and perfectly situated at the bottom of Tasman Bay. To the west are Abel Tasman and Kahurangi National Parks, at least forty by sixty miles of complete wilderness, easily accessible, and perfect for hiking, mountain biking, camping—you name it. I have to say if I were to do this all over, I'd spend the money to rent one of the very nice Mercedes-Benz diesel campers and carry my bike on the back. I saw quite a few of these, and they looked like total heaven as I labored along steep grades, wondering what the hell I was doing.

Tasman Bay is fairly silted, but well protected from the winds and dangerous currents of Cook Strait. The big supertankers have to anchor a ways out, as does any other large ship with a deep draft, but there were long pipes to bring in the oil, and plenty of boats to offload supplies.

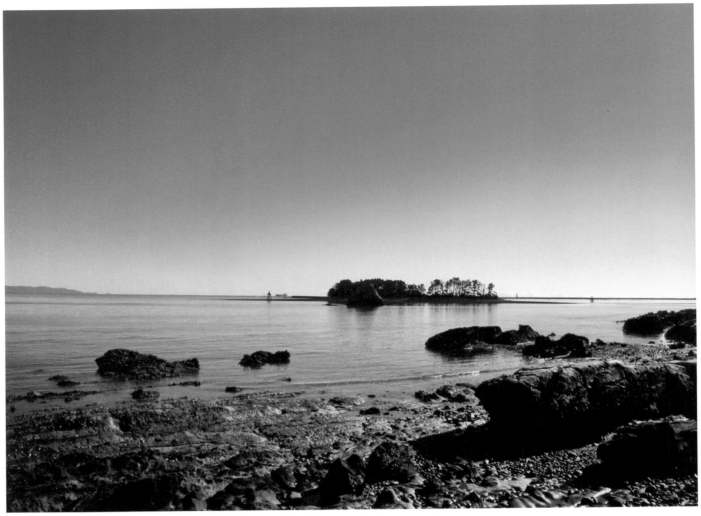

Figure 80 - Tasman Bay. You can just make out an oil tanker moored a long way out

It was here at Nelson I met a man at the backpackers who was an expat American, and he gave me a ton of advice on where to go on the North Island. He suggested I take a two-day rafting/kayaking/canoeing trip down the Whanganui River (remember, the "Wh" is pronounced as an "F"), which he said was an amazing adventure, very beautiful, and a place mostly forgotten by both locals and tourists. It is located in the center of the island, surrounded by national forest, and he pointed out a number of different and easier rides.

I didn't spend more than a day or two in Nelson. It wasn't my gig at the time, and I needed to get my butt east to the ferry back to the North Island to stay on schedule, but I had a couple of really neat rides and places to visit before then. Little did I know the riding was about to get really tough again.

Chapter Nine - Havelock and Kenepuru Sound

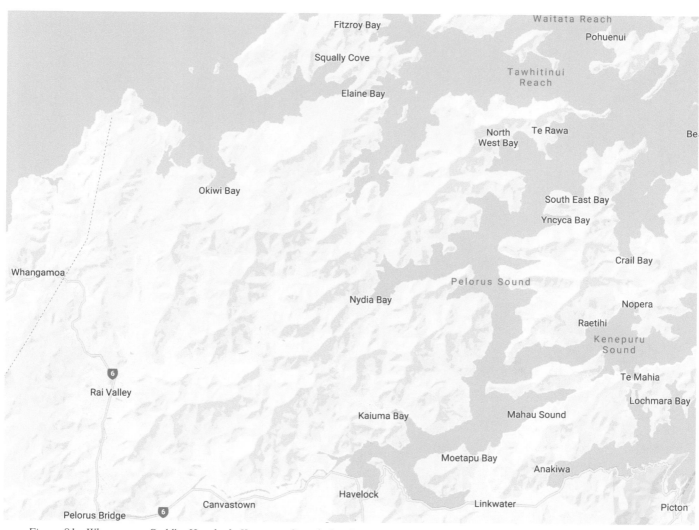

Figure 81 - Whangamoa Saddle, Havelock, Kenepuru Sound, then Picton

I made it up over the Whangamoa Saddle (which along the way transmogrified in my mind to WhackaMoa Saddle), which is a long, eight-kilometer ride up to a height of four hundred meters, followed by a great downhill section, which was a lot of fun indeed, unfortunately followed by another six-kilometer climb up two hundred meters, and yet another thirty-six beyond to Havelock. Ow.

I was going to head on to Picton the following day to catch the ferry, but the next available booking wasn't until Monday due to gale-force winds in the strait. It was Thursday, so I took a boat cruise out into Kenepuru Sound, saw a lot of mussel farms, and got some very nice pics.

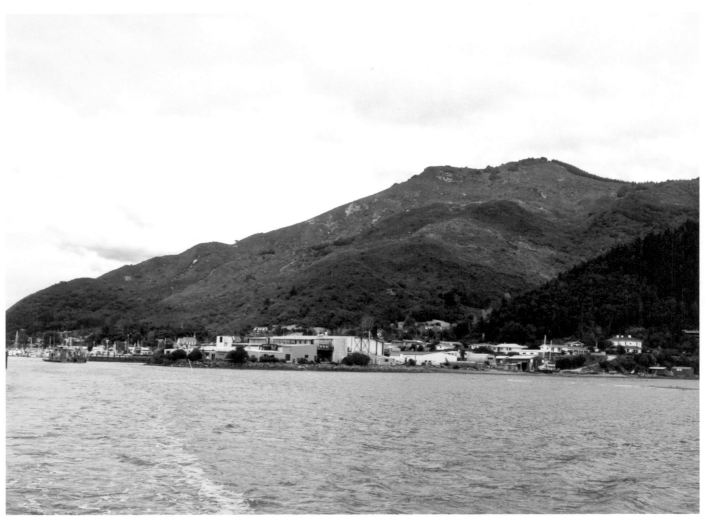

Figure 82 - Kenepuru Sound tour

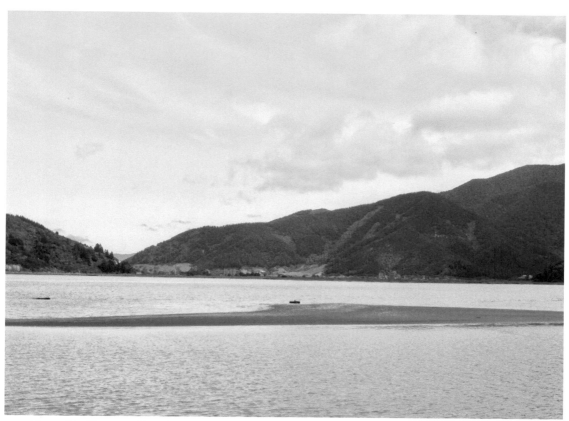

Figure 83 - Kenepuru Sound

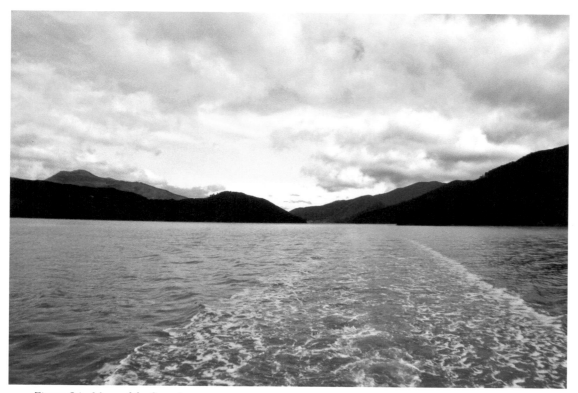

Figure 84 - More of the Sound

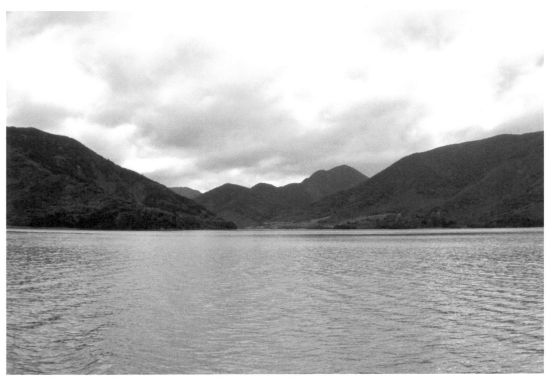

Figure 85 - More of the Sound

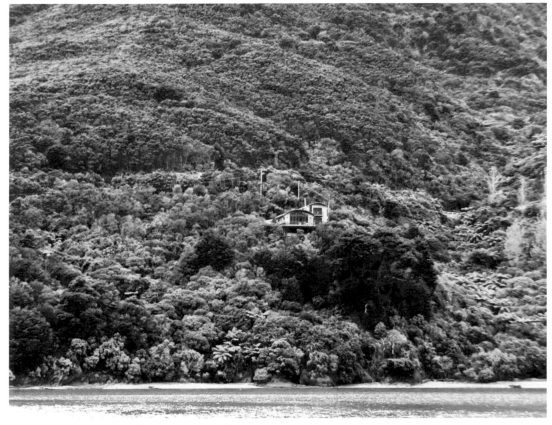

Figure 86 - House with a great view indeed

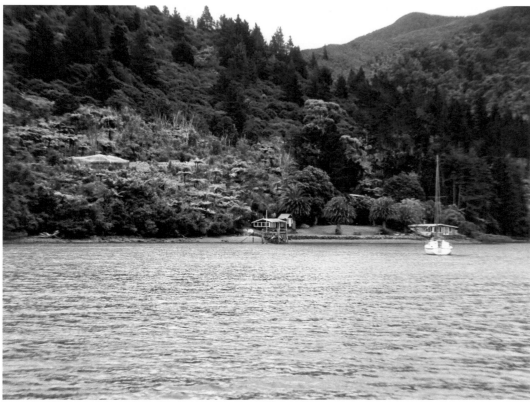

Figure 87 - Another inlet

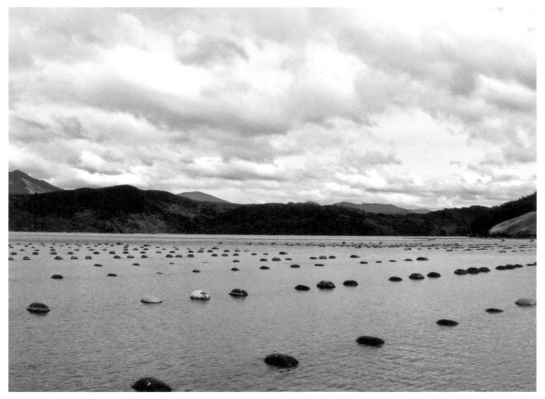

Figure 88 - Oyster farm

That evening I enjoyed some karaoke with the locals at the Slip Inn (which isn't an inn, but a hotel/café/bar right on the water). It was nice to be able to concentrate only on vocals and not have to play guitar at the same time and attempt some tunes I'd never sung before. I pulled off a reasonable version of "Please Come to Boston" by Kenny Loggins, "I Can't Tell You Why" by The Eagles, and a couple of others. All was had by a good time.

I took a couple of days to head out on a peninsula, along Kenepuru Road that meanders along the coast and bays and inlets, with the destination being Portage. BTW, if you're interested, along this entire distance there's a walking/hiking path called the Queen Charlotte Track.

But good ol' Murphy struck again. He's such a friendly fellow, coming around so often. The "easy" forty-kilometer ride out to Portage turned out to be every bit as hard as the WhackaMoa Saddle: steep ups and downs for twenty-five kilometers straight. I met a fellow cyclist whose rig consisted of a road-bike style (I still call 'em ten-speeds), but she was also towing a two-wheeled contraption that was basically a large storage box on wheels. She was pushing the rig up one of the hills, as was I. I didn't feel quite so bad thereafter, nor so alone in the world. It was raining constantly, but that was most welcome given the level of effort.

I stayed the night at the Te Mahia Bay resort near Portage, an upscale place, very nice, with a spa (hot tub) and sauna that felt like heaven on earth. There was a celebration in the hotel for a lady turning eighty (didn't look it!). Sitting down waiting for my turn in the restaurant, it came to the attention of another US expat that I was American, and then came a barrage of questions I was happy to answer. But I learned something interesting: he said that Kiwiland had changed significantly over the past thirty years. It was a truly different land back then, but now he feels that if he moved back to Portland (Oregon), the culture shock would be minimal. Apparently New Zealand had "upgraded" itself to the twentieth century, and Auckland likes to push its politics on everyone. I doubted if that was a good thing, and whether the locals agreed. Apparently the economy was better. The West Coast on the South Island was considered the last vestige of true Kiwiland, as it's fairly isolated, with very few roads.

The next day, on the way back, I noticed my legs were definitely getting stronger. My riding was better too: I was shifting gears at the right time, I was leaning into the turns better, my pedaling circles (ellipses, really) were consistent, and I could time my acceleration of down the slopes and the following hike up the next hill so as to ease the overall effort. My hamstrings were getting into the fun as well, as I could pull myself along now. It was a new sensation.

I grabbed a few more pics of Havelock before leaving, including a rare Ferrari, a beautiful, large tree of unknown species, and one with the fog settling in over the town, before riding on to Picton.

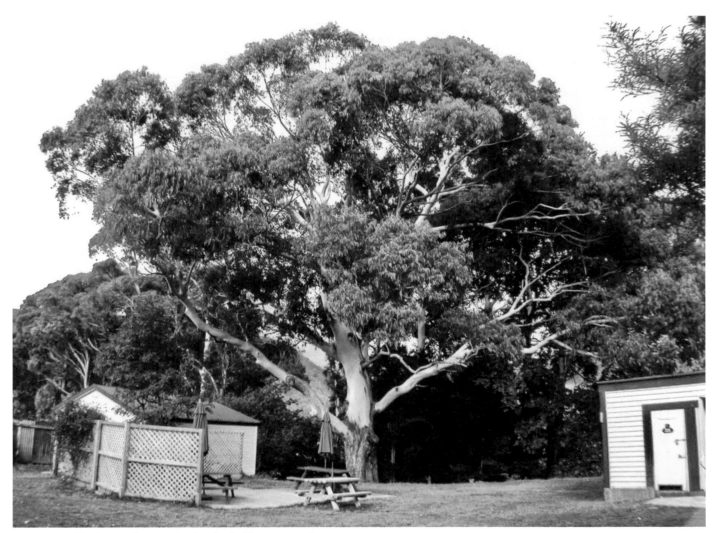

Figure 89 - Unusual tree with white bark. This one caught my eye.

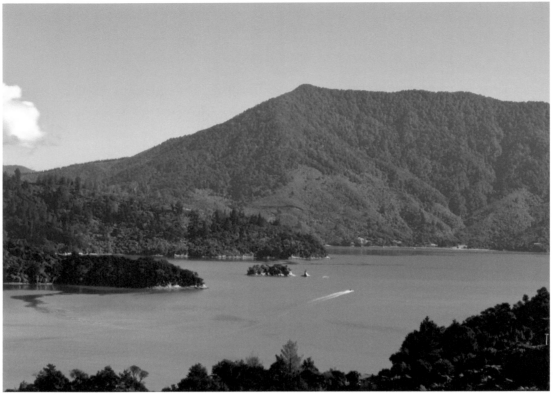

Figure 90 - Heading towards Picton now - a view from the roadside

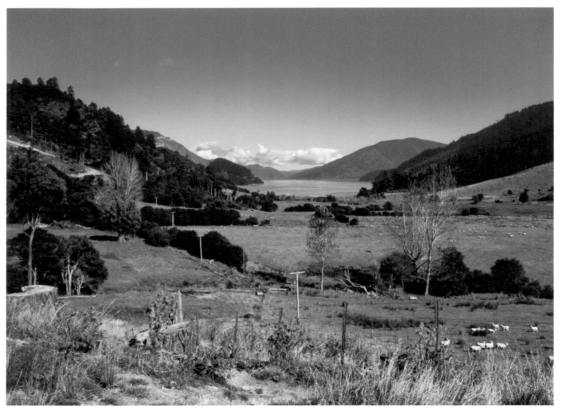

Figure 91 - Serene and pretty

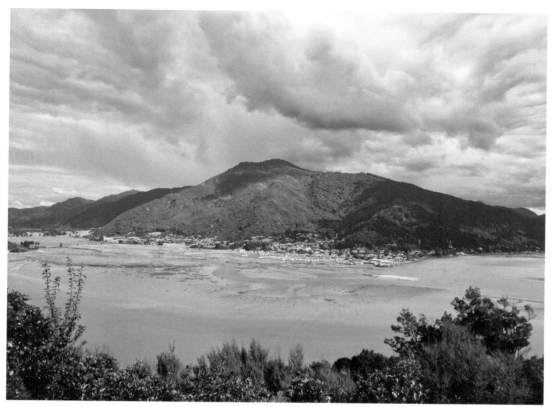

Figure 92 - A view back at Havelock

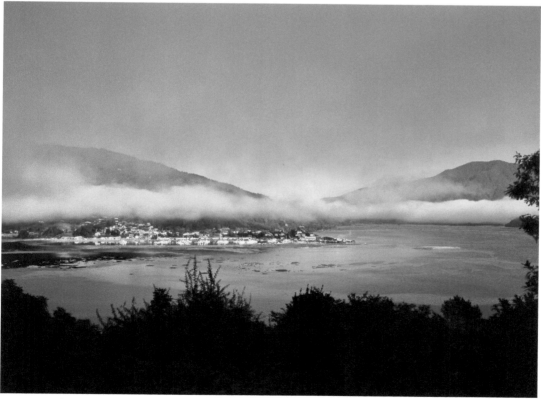

Figure 93 - Fog over the town

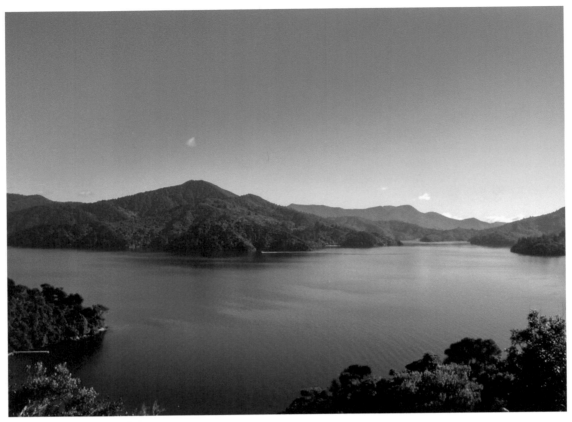

Figure 94 - Towards Picton

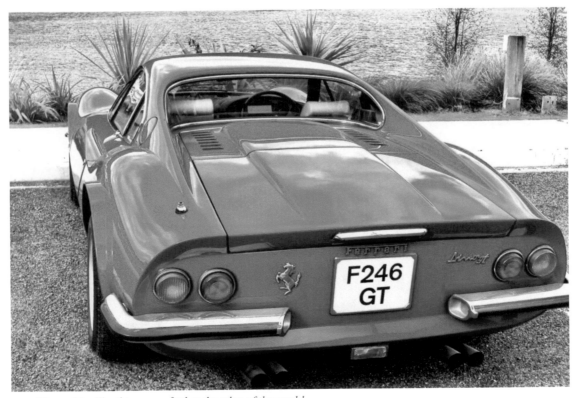

Figure 95 - The things you find at the edge of the world

I had one more hard little slog (a great Kiwi word) over to Picton to catch the 9:30 a.m. ferry. Along the way I greeted a fellow during one of my frequent "walks" (er, of pushing the bike up a steep slope), whose daughters were in the US, one of whom was a model (ahem, unfortunately married). These kinds of casual conversations with a complete stranger are the norm in New Zealand. All in all a very friendly, laid-back bunch.

I was looking forward now to giving my legs a break, to kick back, do some kayaking, and be more of a tourist. Kiwi was starting to take over my brain—I could almost understand rugby! I could just about translate a heavy Kiwi accent, though it still took a second or two.

I did get one nice picture of the town of Picton from above, looking down into the harbor, before jumping the ferry.

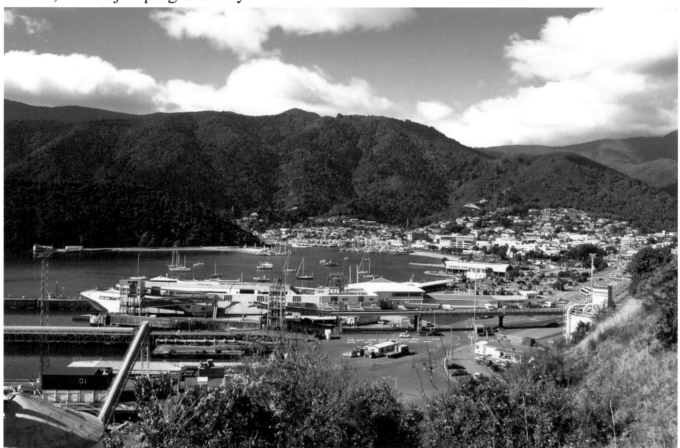

Figure 96 - Picton Harbor

Chapter Ten - The Whanganui River Trip

In Wellington I had a bit more time to explore the town before taking the bus on to my next destination. The south arm of the starfish-shaped North Island wanders a bit southwest, and Wellington is located at the tip, inside a bay with a southern opening. It's well protected, with a half-moon crest of hills to the west. There's a good walking area in the town center full of shops and a great museum of the native peoples. It's a more real New Zealand town than Auckland will ever be.

From Wellington to Auckland it's twelve hours by train, but I exited halfway up at the little village of National Park. The rail bisects the North Island before heading off northwest. To the right as you travel along are big, quiet volcanos (for the most part—one blew its top in '95). The middle of the island is wide open, with large vistas, rolling hills, and empty country. I didn't get to the west coast, or the east coast; I understand the former is extremely difficult riding, with constant ups and downs, while the latter is quite lush with great farm-to-table restaurants, when you can find them, and wonderful cattle country as well.

National Park is comprised of a couple hotels, a backpackers, one tavern, and one gas station/food shop. It truly is in the middle of nowhere. There I booked a three-day trip down the Whanganui River.

It was dicey proposition from the start: I told the guy I had no camping gear. "Oh, well, you can just borrow my sleeping bag." "Will I need food?" "Yes, you'll have to provide all of your own food." What the hell was I getting myself into?

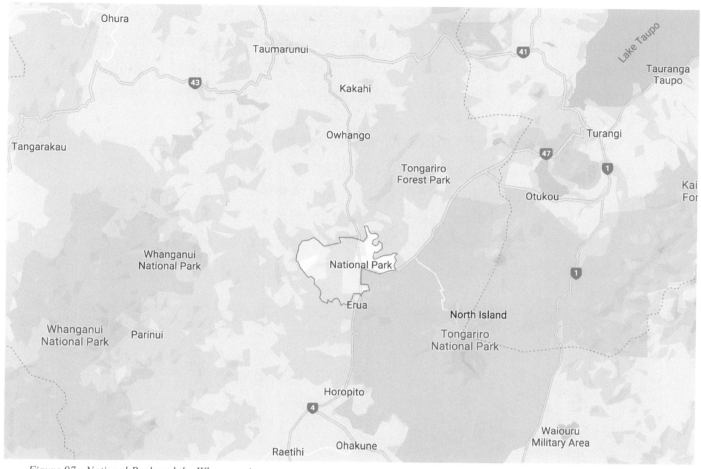

Figure 97 - National Park and the Whanganui

I was expecting a guided tour, and a light workout while floating along downstream, but Murphy struck again. Apparently this fellow I booked with tends, in the words of the gentlemen staffing the counter at the National Park backpackers, "to kind of miss some things, or forgets to mention others."

I was dropped off on the banks of the river, with almost no food, no equipment to cook food with if I so wished (he was vague on this, as he said I could borrow his gear, but I never did find his gear, so . . .), along with a choice of two lousy kayaks. Not true river kayaks, but kind of inbetweeners, with no back support and slow as molasses in winter. The two German girls I was dropped off with wanted to be left alone in their own world, so there I was. I lost the map almost right away, of course, though thankfully I found it later on the next day.

The Whanganui River is in the middle-west section and is very, very remote. It's also a proper river, not like those "streams" we have out in Colorado. Pictures don't do it justice. There are numerous inlets that break out into little waterfalls, lush tropical plants, and thick moss, and I also spotted an unusual-looking hawk. After the first night of constant paddling (the river was low that year), my back was in so much pain I was willing to cut the trip short and go back, but there was no way out - not even a trail - and the bush was too dense to navigate.

I had always been really inflexible. I was one of those kids that could never sit cross-legged (I can now, though not comfortably), and it was very painful for me to do any kind of stretching (and still is). I thought it was that way for everyone. Not so! Anyway, really stiff hamstrings didn't allow me to lean forward enough to take the pressure off of my lower back. As a result (and I should have known), kayaking is a big no-no for me. Canoeing might have been a better choice.

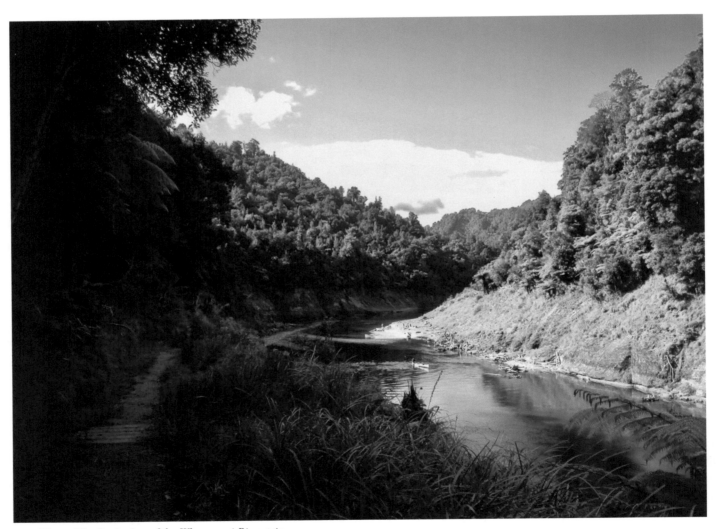

Figure 98 - Beginning of the Whanganui River trip

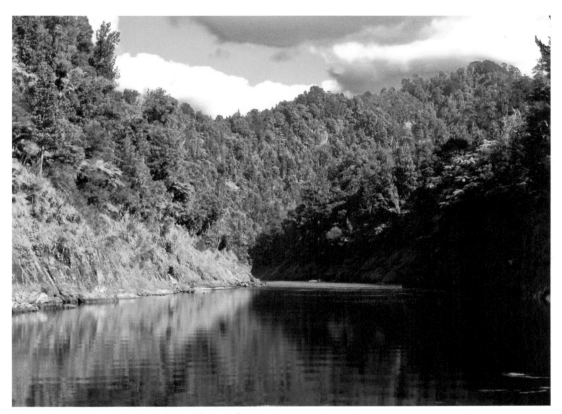

Figure 99 - The river was low and quiet that year

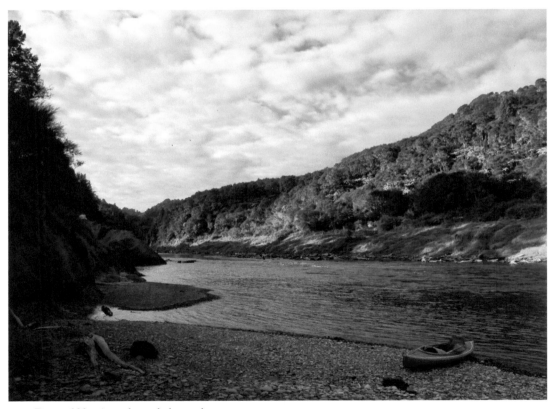

Figure 100 - A much needed stretch

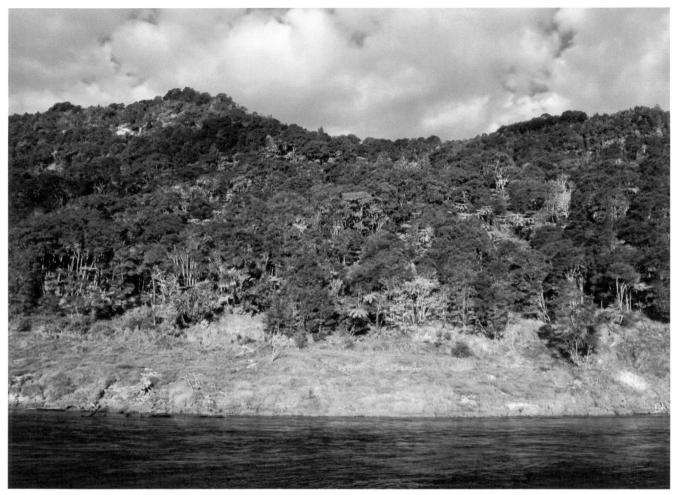

Figure 101 - It was eerily quiet as there were almost no birds due to a possum invasion

There are really two kinds of tours to do on the river: one with the Maori, staying at one of their *mawaes*, a long, lodge-type building that reminds me of the Iroquois. One must be invited to stay at a mawae. The other way is via Kiwi tour guide. I ended up sort of tagging along with the latter, a proper crew of about twenty-two people with two guides, after meeting them at the first overnight stop.

This place only had a "hut" (owned by the Department of Conservancy) with no amenities: no hot water, no showers, a gas stove, and a gas heater (both of these set low to conserve gas). Shivering, fresh off the river, my feet numb, and soaked to the bone, I was considering what torture technique to use on the man who got me into this mess: slow-turning spit over an open fire, or bamboo shoots under the fingernails?

I re-rigged the boat in the morning, giving myself more lower back support. About halfway through the day (still tagging along with the tour group), we all stopped to take a break and anchored where there were some good hiking trails, even one up to the infamous Bridge to Nowhere.

The story goes that after WWI the government gave some land up here in the boonies to returning soldiers, should they be so inclined to have it, with the hope this would lead to more permanent settlements. Unfortunately, the only "road" into the area was the river, and rivers are, well, alive, fickle, and do their own thing. By the thirties this effort had failed, with the last remnants of humanity walking off the land, leaving everything behind.

The bridge is a very well-done, short concrete bridge. I took some nice pictures on the hike up and back (but not of the bridge itself, oddly enough). The trail does in fact continue after the bridge for some kilometers, to no city or town anywhere. It seemed an attractive option to explore. Who knows what one might really find?

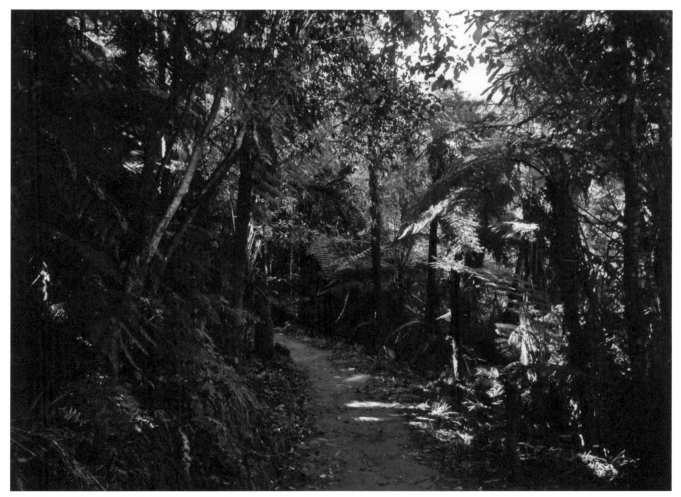

Figure 102 - Path to the Bridge to Nowhere

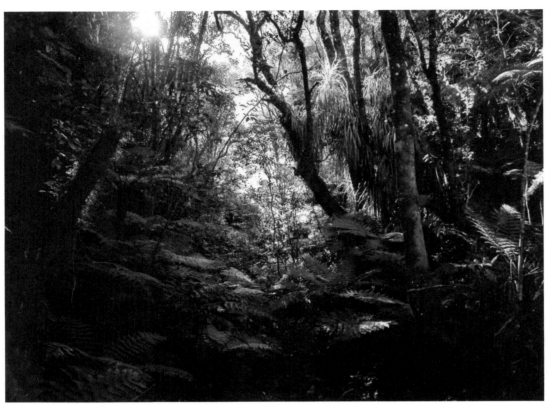

Figure 103 - More North island jungle

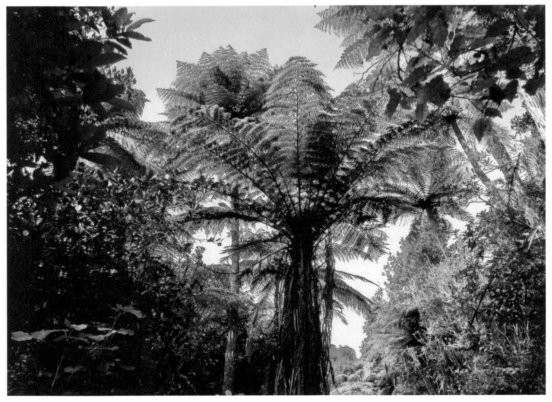

Figure 104 - Tall pretty trees

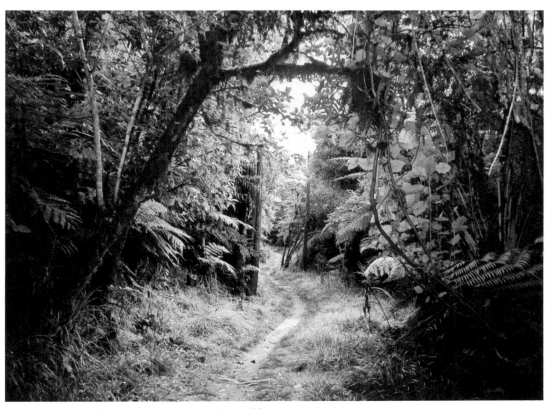

Figure 105 - What mysteries lie along this path?

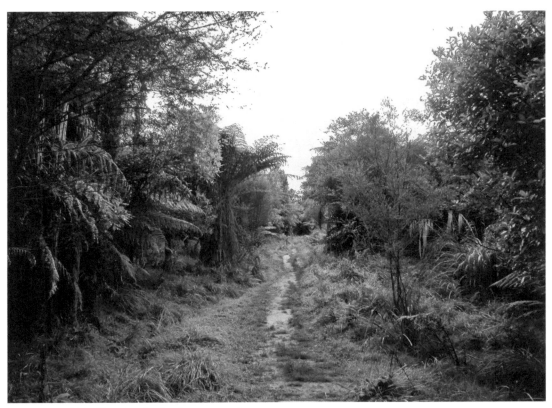

Figure 106 - There's a bridge here, somewhere

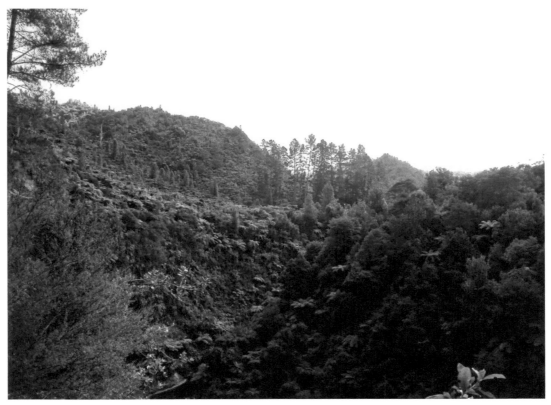

Figure 107 - From the bridge, looking...south?

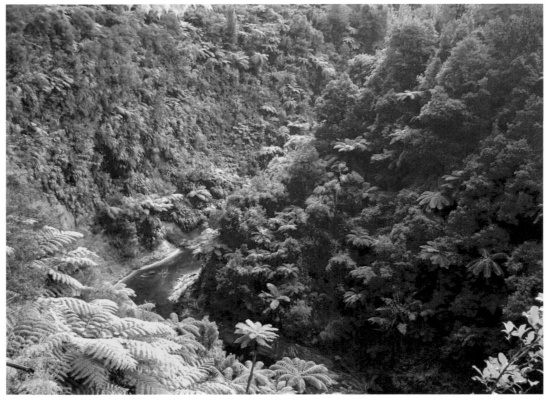

Figure 108 - From the bridge looking down at one of the tributaries

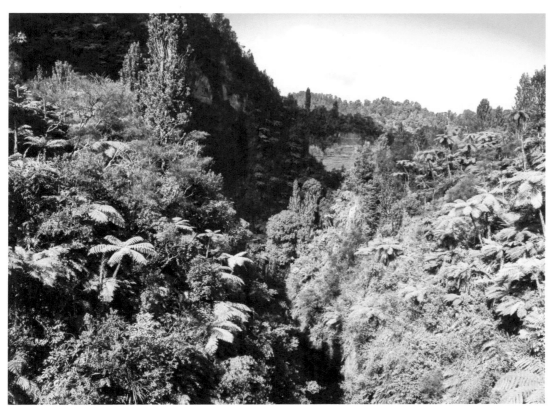

Figure 109 - Old cliffs, covered in foliage

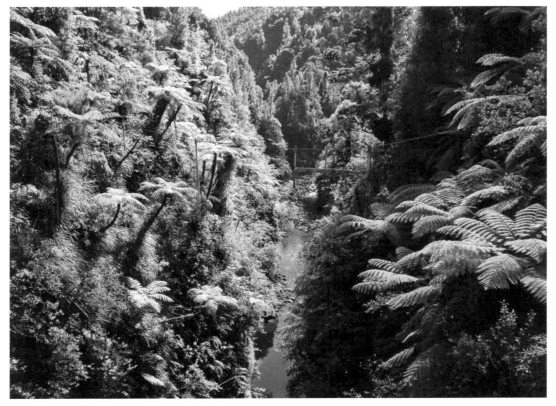

Figure 110 - Remains of a wooden bridge

We met another guide downriver that was conducting another kind of tour—this time on a jet boat, a very high horsepower thingamajob that flies along the surface of the water. I'd seen them back in Queenstown, and at least four different ones in my travels through this country. They typically did double duty by rescuing stranded/dumped/drowning people. I got to ride on one later the next day.

Anyway, this fellow told me that at the end of the day's journey we'd end up at Joe's Lodge, where I could stay if I liked, for NZ$75, and get a hot shower, a real place to sleep, dinner, and breakfast. Sold, done deal!

Joe's Lodge, a.k.a. the Ramanui Lodge, was a wonderful place, with a friendly pig who walked up to everyone, plopped down on his side, and expected to be scratched. There were also a few dogs, a rambunctious kitten, chickens, a rooster, and a couple of very happy horses that were content to be ridden bareback but mostly just appreciated the attention.

The landing at the river was difficult going. There wasn't much purchase, and a strong current kept pulling you away, but the jet boat pulled up alongside, and I managed with their help. Turned out I missed the first landing, and it wouldn't be the last time I missed such a thing.

I was cold, again, and my feet and legs didn't want to respond, but I changed into dry clothes and started feeling better in a hurry. I should say that included with my kayak was a couple of small barrels where one can store gear. They are supposedly waterproof, though I found the next day that wasn't quite the case. I took a picture from the lodge at dusk that is still my favorite from all my travels in New Zealand. It's the one where you can just make out the sign saying Ramanui Lodge.

The timing was good: hot shower, good food, good people. I slept hard.

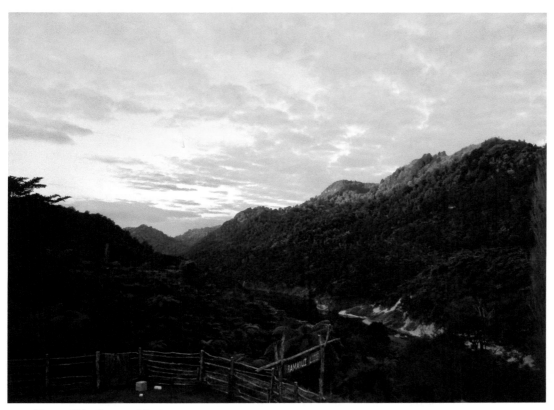

Figure 111 - Ramanui Lodge

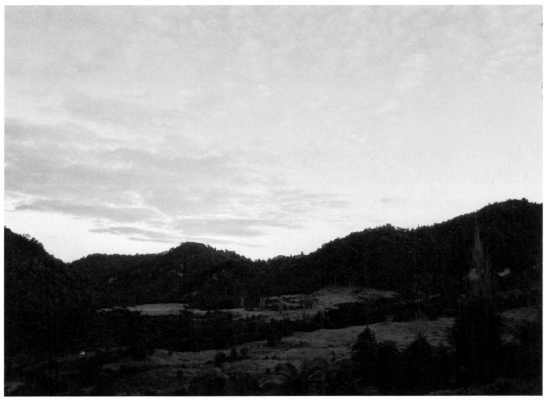

Figure 112 - From the lodge, looking south

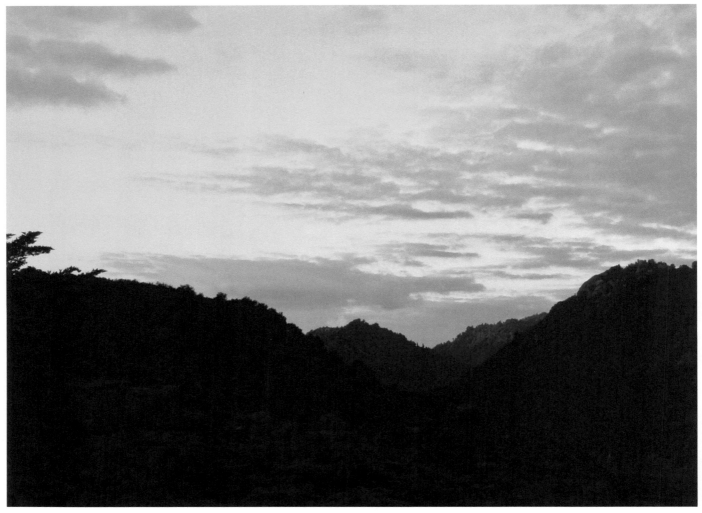

Figure 113 - Sunset. Warm, wonderful.

The weather the next day was just gorgeous. I can thank my Dad for my warm-bloodedness, as I actually like humidity, as long as it stays in the eighties or so. There was no rain, just a mist that covered everything until the sun burned it off around mid-morning.

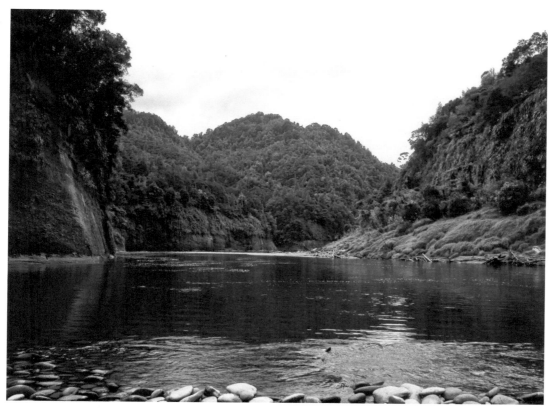

Figure 114 - Back on the quiet Whanganui

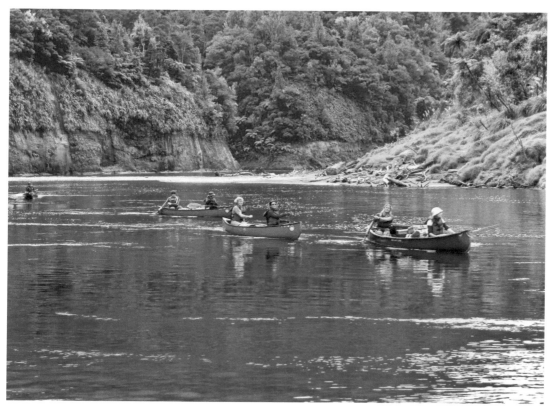

Figure 115 - The tour I tagged along with

My pace slowed considerably, and I let others take the lead. After a while, having lost sight of the group, I came upon a bunch of them stopped on the side of the river. They were all contemplating some grade two rapids up ahead. Naturally, they invited me to go ahead of them, probably so they could just point and laugh.

I didn't know, and they didn't tell me, that the first two groups through had been dumped unceremoniously by the waters (though rescued by an awaiting jet boat), and they graciously allowed me to let me go next (yeah, right). Paddling hard I almost made it through, but at the last moment, just when I thought I had made it to safety, a big wave rose up out of nowhere, slapped me on the left side, and up and over I went.

Lost my damn glasses too. I had forgotten they were even on. The barrels appeared to stay sealed and were picked up by the jet boat along with me and the rest of the floating debris. My camera did make it through unscathed, having been in a barrel, avoiding what moisture did make it in, but I was blowing river water out of my nose the rest of the day.

The others coming downstream wisely stayed far to the left, which was the safe thing to do, and made it around the rapids just fine. The rest of the day was short, and I ended my three-day journey at Papiriki (which translates to "Paprika" for those of us trying to remember strange Maori names).

Of course, the sign on the shore for the landing to Papiriki was the size of a postage stamp, so I missed it. About four kilometers downriver I started getting that nasty little feeling inside that something was very wrong, so I moored my kayak in a muddy bank and hiked up a dirt road. I was fortunate and got a ride from another crazy Kiwi driver and found out the truth about that landing. I felt quite foolish when I had to ask Joe for a ride back downstream to retrieve my stuff.

Chapter Eleven - Lake Taupo and Whakatane

Back at National Park, I decided to stay another night just to recover. It was now Tuesday, April 16, 2002. I left the next day for a fifty-kilometer "flat ride with a hill at the end," which by now you can guess actually means in Kiwi "steeply rolling hills with a thousand-foot climb."

Several thoughts occurred to me on this ride. "Kiwis really need to build more shoulders on their roads," and "If I mounted a submachine gun on the front and fired at the idiots who flew by me with only a couple feet to spare, would anyone really care?" And I decided that Bill D. Cat had the perfect description for climbing steep hills: "Ack. Gag. Barf."

My eyes were doing pretty well, sans glasses. One doesn't travel too fast on a bike anyway, so I had plenty of time to read the signs. I ended up going without for the rest of the trip, and after the several days of the initial angst, forgot they were even missing.

Tongariro National Park was to the south as I traveled, home of Mount Tongariro which blew its top in 2012, and the area I was in now was near the big volcanic plateau. It had some amazing scenery: open vistas, shortish trees, windy, and this part of the road did indeed have a shoulder! On the backside of my little mountain climb, I hit 69 kph going downhill. That was quite a ride! I was already at a fair elevation—National Park is at 825 meters, or about twenty-four hundred feet, so I had quite a distance to get back down.

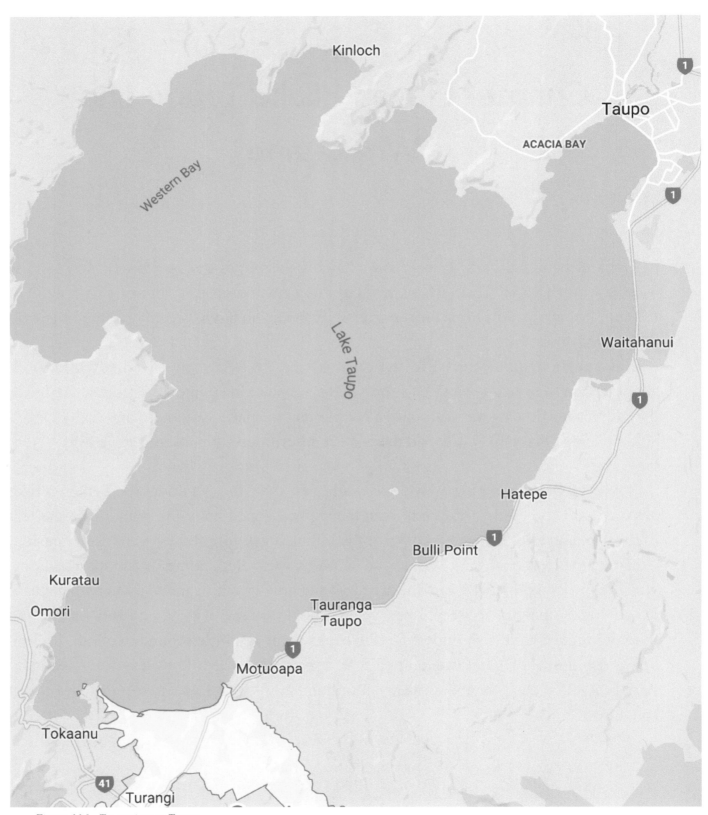

Figure 116 - Turangi up to Taupo

I was planning to stay the night at Extreme Backpackers in Turangi, a town at the south end of Lake Taupo, and the self-proclaimed "Trout Capital of New Zealand." I stopped at the information center (all towns in Kiwiland seem to have them—very useful things), and the woman told me, "You're looking for Extreme Backpackers? Oh no! That's way over in Taumarunui, which is 150k away." She was pulling my leg, you see, but that's typical of the Kiwi humor. The backpackers was only one block down the street.

But I now had a feeling deep down inside after the river trip that I was getting burned out. Too much traveling, not enough vacationing. I headed north along the east side of Lake Taupo, hit another steep hill, and then made it to the town of Taupo at the northeast end of the lake.

I still remember this part, being on the side of the road, resting my legs, looking back at the lake. I was allowing the truckers to go by (there was a shoulder, but it wasn't super wide), and with two lanes going uphill, one for passing, and plenty of traffic it could make their life difficult to pass a cyclist. They usually gave me a honk in appreciation when I pulled over.

Some little notes to catch up on: I passed 1,000k for the trip at the crest of the little "hill" going into Turangi. I had done about 950k on the South Island. My belt was finally willing to be tightened a notch, and my legs were feeling pretty good, all things considered.

This area is the big ultramarathoners/distance runners/mountain bikers paradise for the North Island, as Queenstown is for the South. But the feeling was completely different: a bit more crowded, and a lingering sense of doom. Lake Taupo itself is one big-ass caldera created by a supervolcano approximately twenty-six thousand years ago (see yer local Wikipedia entry). The entire area is, needless to say, still active.

I took a few very nice pictures around Lake Taupo, including one of the infamous black swan—a pair of them, in fact. They're apparently like our Canadian geese, a real pest. Hard to believe, but true.

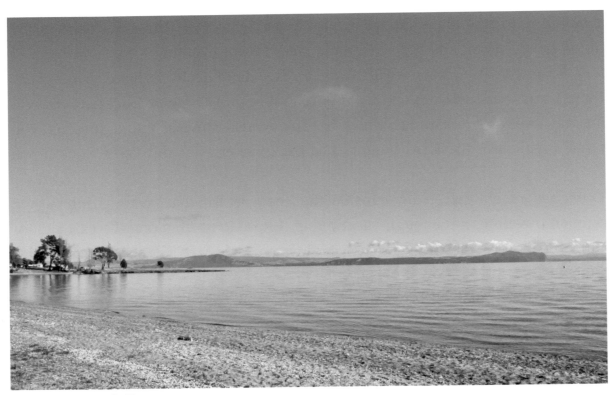

Figure 117 - Lake Taupo

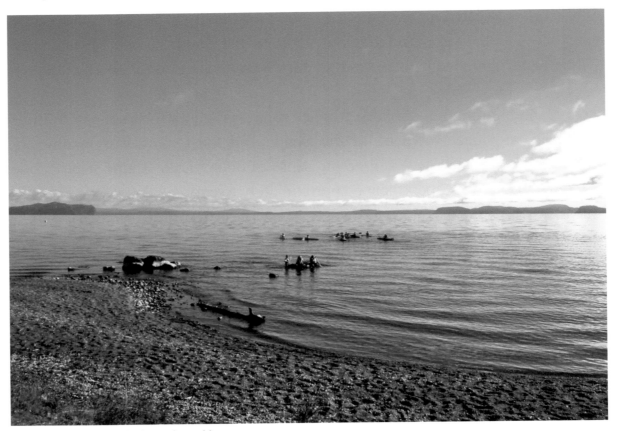

Figure 118 - Yes, that's one big caldera

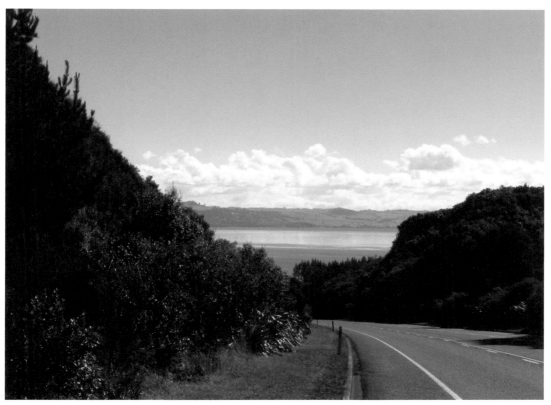

Figure 119 - Off the side of the road, looking back at the lake

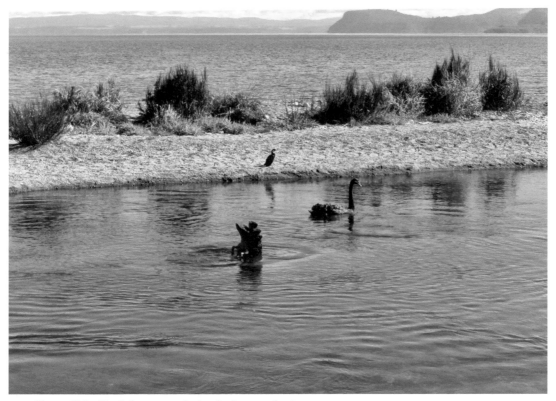

Figure 120 - Black Swans, no doubt plotting our demise

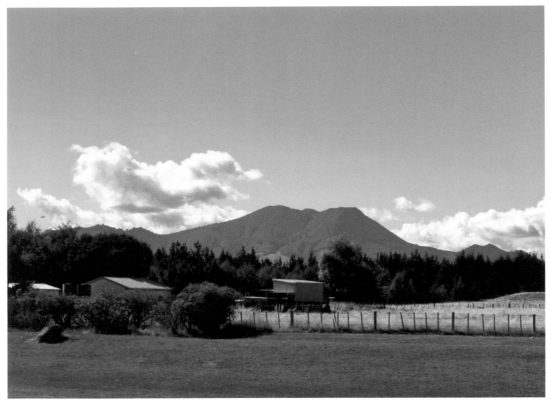

Figure 121 - One of the many extinct volcanos in the area

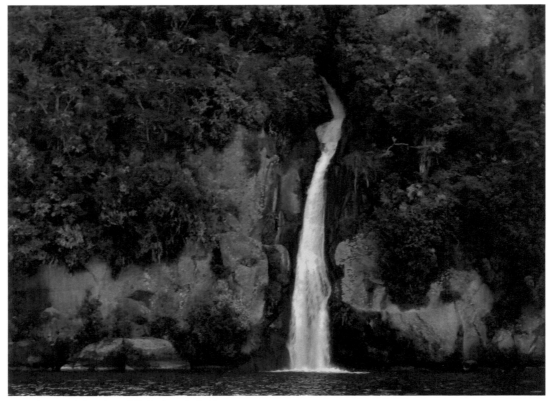

Figure 122 - Waterfall feeding Lake Taupo

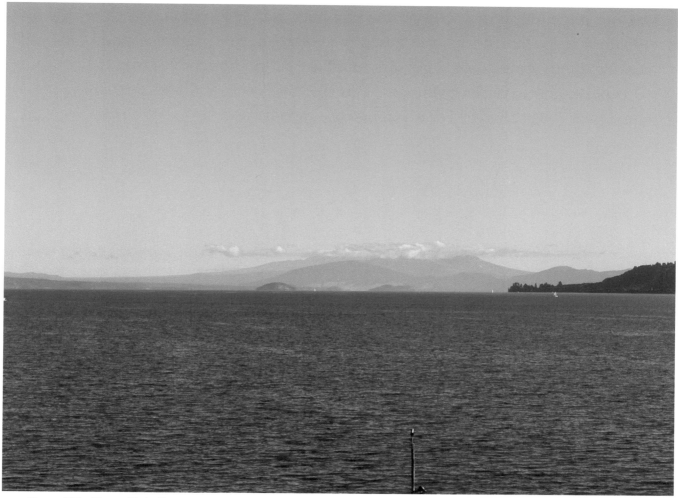

Figure 123 - More of Lake Taupo

I stayed in the area for almost a week, resting, visiting hot tubs, and even got a massage. For those that are wondering, no, I didn't get "lucky" on this trip. I wasn't exactly feeling well and didn't have much energy in the evenings to drink beer and chase women. This would continue for several years after which I started dating. One was a very nice, professional woman living in the Virginia area for a bit, but originally from Bangor, Maine. But the late nights out with her drained me silly, and I had to call it off. Too bad; she was special. You would have thought my now I would've gotten professional help (for my physical problems, at the least), but no. But I guess I must have been feeling better when in the fall of 2005 (back when I was still chasing the dragon for those who are familiar with the phrase) I met my ex-wife-to-be.

I was officially burned out from riding at this point. So I jumped a bus down to Whakatane via Rotorua to visit the only currently (at that time) active volcano, which

113

was out on White Island. During the two-hour stop at Rotorua, I took a little look around: it was a tourist trap, and I didn't like it at all. Not that there weren't the usual amazing things to see, such as geysers, mudflats, sulfuric creeks, orgasmic trout fishing, wild forest, and towering palms. It's just that the locals had sold everything for the tourist buck. Okay, maybe I was just in a bad mood.

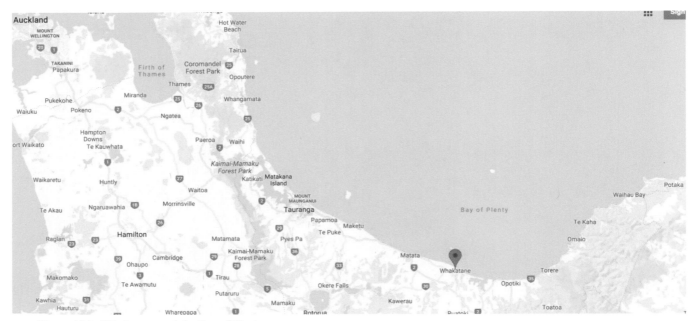

Figure 124 - Whakatane and the Bay of Plenty

Whakatane is great: it's a laid-back, Southern California-style town under some cliffs and right on the water, on the south end of the Bay of Plenty. At thirty-seven degrees south, the climate is perfect.

I stayed at the Whakatane Hotel, which also included the Craic Irish Pub. As the front desk area was undergoing repairs, I checked in at the pub, where I was branded a "Canadian," and then in a spat of revisionist history, the bartender corrected her story to "American." Stinkin' Kiwis. But boy didn't I fall in love right away: she was a short, beautiful brunette with that wonderful sing-song Kiwi accent, and damn it to hell, she was happily married.

The hotel was a somewhat quaint, personable place with scripted glass in the bathroom doors, pipes that rumble and moan, yet everything had a clean and fresh feeling, probably due to the wonderful air that permeated everything.

I walked along the downtown area looking for an internet shop to send off an email and found a café/sandwich place called Friends. (As of this writing it appears to no longer be in existence.) Smooth jazz was playing in the background, and a couple of expats were hanging out talking about the Saints NFL draft picks (to which I immediately corrected the name to The Ain'ts), and the proprietor, clearly an expat himself, looked like he was from Southern California and knew a whole lot of Jimmy Buffet.

The following morning found me on that ferry, waiting to head out to White Island, listening to Robbie Williams, and actually feeling good for once.

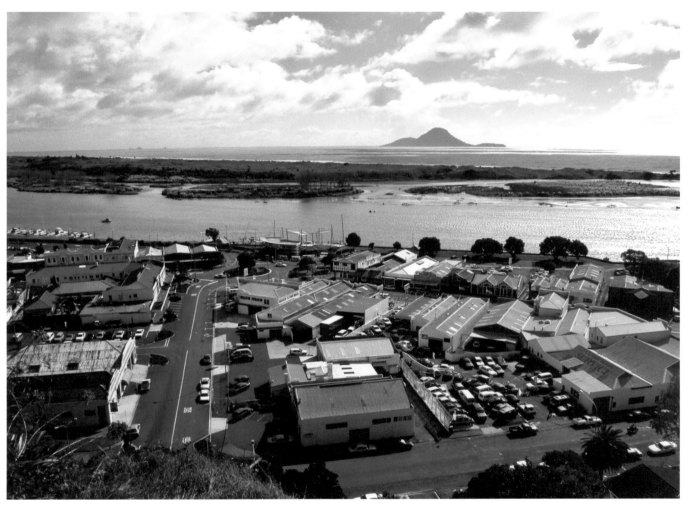

Figure 125 - Whakatane at last! With White Island in the distance

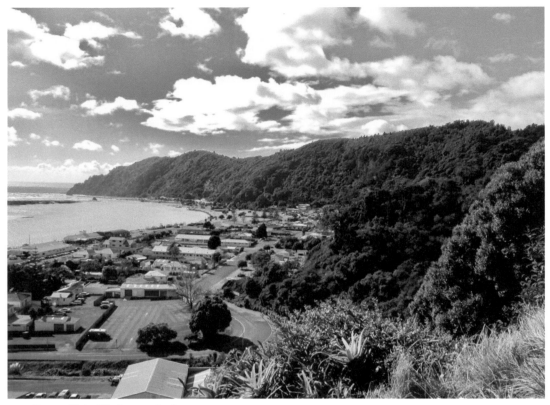

Figure 126 - Whakatane, looking east

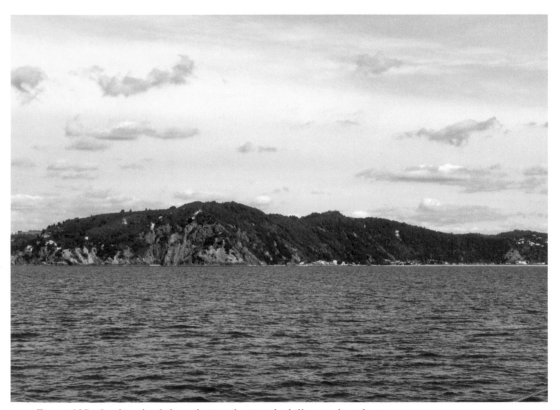

Figure 127 - Looking back from the tour boat at the hills guarding the town

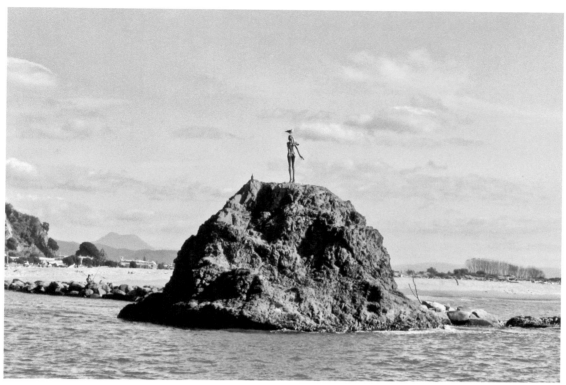

Figure 128 - At the mouth of the inlet to Whakatane harbor

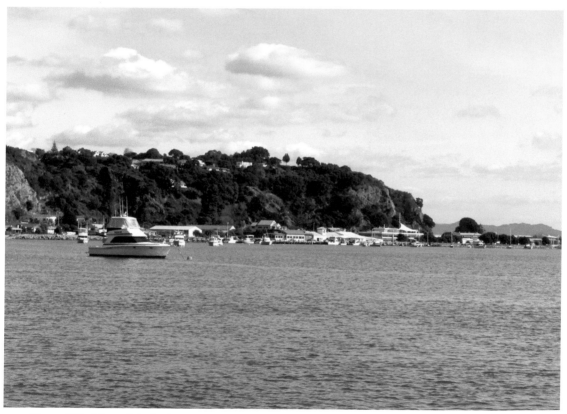

Figure 129 - More of the harbor

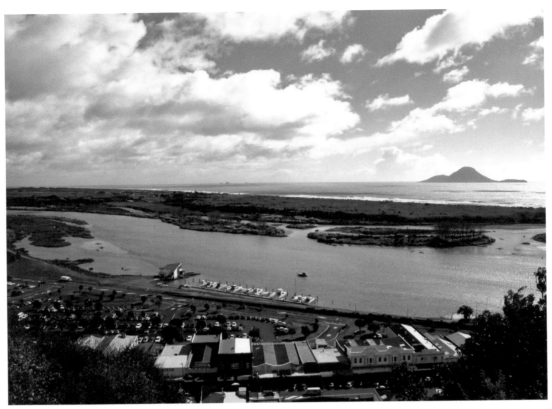

Figure 130 - Another view from above

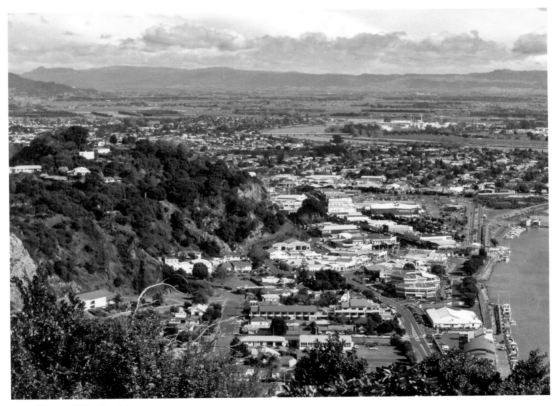

Figure 131 - Looking west.

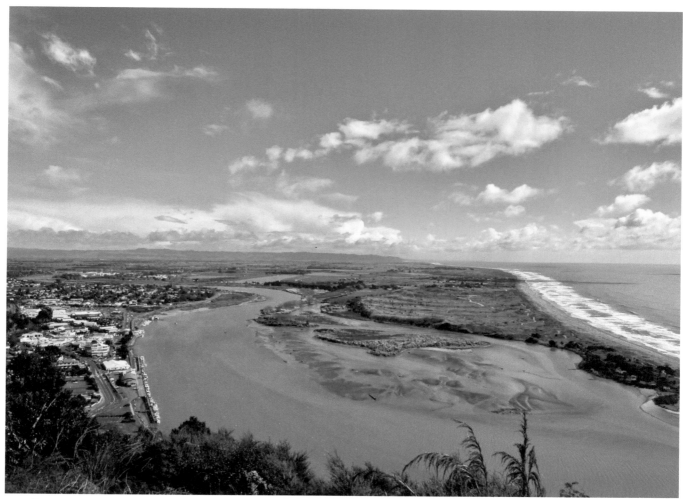

Figure 132 - Another view, northwest towards Auckland

Chapter Twelve - What It's All About

Lyme is a bitch of a disease, especially after fifty years. My doctor, Dr. Bill Billica, said I probably caught it around the age of seven, which just so happens was right when my personality and behavior changed so drastically. This answered many, many questions. When he told me the prognosis, I immediately burst out in tears: I just *knew* it to be the truth.

Anyway, this means I got the disease back in 1968, years before it was even discovered. I had all of the classic symptoms: bad memory, poor concentration and mind fog, depression, withdrawal, feeling of being isolated (cue Pink Floyd's "The Wall," which is no joke), lack of coordination, chronic fatigue syndrome, a bad case of constipation, and more. But had you told me any time along the way that I had Lyme, I would have thought you were crazy. Perspective is indeed a bitch.

I mean, I never went to see a doctor complaining of symptoms, because I thought everything was okay; you know, normal wear and tear. And the only reason I even went to get checked in the first place was because a friend of mine, who had three times the troubles I was experiencing, had recommended it, otherwise I would have just kept on going, not knowing. We men (I can only speak for us) are pretty amazingly adaptable and tough, or can be, and we readily put the needs of others before ourselves, especially when it comes to loved ones and family. So, pain gets put in the background. This approach works for a while until one gets behind on the maintenance. Like an older car, if you don't keep up, things start to break, and then it can get really expensive and time consuming to fix.

As I write this, seventeen years later now, I am free and clear. I believe the die-off was the Wednesday before Thanksgiving of 2018, but the official word came a few weeks later. My doctor is an M.D. but has developed a program using more natural ingredients. It was a long, seven-month process that was worse than the disease but achieved without heavy antibiotics (thankfully). Lyme is quite expert at hiding from the immune system using something called a "bio film", but his approach breaks that down as well so *all* of the little suckers can be killed.

It also turned out that I had been infected at the same time with the non-STD version of chlamydia. Yeah, like who would have known there was such a thing? This was cause of my inflexibility as it attacks and scars the fascia, which is a sort of Saran wrap around the muscles, greatly restricting range of motion.

I had also picked up a bad case of mycoplasma (walking pneumonia) within the last few years, which really weakened my lungs, so I had to kill off these two infections first before I could even tackle the Lyme, and these little suckers fought back *hard*. Turns out they fight back harder and harder until the final die-off. The chlamydia started restricting my movement so greatly that one night it took substantial concentrated mental efforts to lift my right arm over my head. It didn't hurt, mind you, it just didn't want to move.

And boy were my lungs a mess - back in that February I drove up to meet some friends in Rocky Mountain National Park for a few hours of snowshoeing. I planned carefully - I even stayed in Estes Park the previous night in order to allow me to acclimate to the higher altitude (I live at 6,000 feet, so you'd think I'd already be accustomed to the thinner air, but I was being extra careful). Despite this, the following morning as I drove up and into the park I started having serious problems, first gasping for air, unable to catch my breath, then I started to black out - not a joyful thing to happen while driving. Needless to say I quickly turned around and called it a day.

You have to understand that this scared me silly. My father died of a degenerative lung disease back in 2004 - I saw him pass right in front of me, gasping horribly for any kind of breath. I sent my mom out of the room so she wouldn't have to deal with it, did what I was told by the folks manning the phones at 911, and attempted to revive him to no avail. Not a fun day.

Then a year later my brother passed from lymphoma. It was under control until they over-radiated his lungs accidentally, and that was that. It turned out I didn't get to see him before he passed - I guess I was spared by the forces that be another traumatic episode, as he and I were quite close.

Thankfully after that episode, in a couple of months I was able to handle a trip to altitude pretty well. Though there was an initial panic, a friend, bless him, calmed me down and I made it through just fine. Since the mycoplasma died, I haven't had another incident, and my lungs have slowly regained their strength. Cross yer fingers, knock on wood…

There are a number of other bacteria that can live in the belly of a tick and can infect you along with the Lyme (its medical name is *Borrelia*). There's about a 50 percent co-infection rate, with a 30 percent chance of two or more. So besides the chlamydia, you can get infected by such wonderful little buggers as *Babesia*, which is a malaria-type infection; *Rickettsia*, which runs from mild to fatal; *Bartonella, Ehrlichia*, and *Anaplasma*, among others.

As for *Borrelia*, there are over one hundred different species worldwide, including a strain in Japan and even one in the Black Forest of Germany. Rocky Mountain Spotted Fever is a variant as well.

Besides the chronic fatigue, memory loss, and other joys, one can add the aforementioned tendency to run away from problems (also known as the fight or flight syndrome). I figure it this way: your body is fighting a major infection, so something always feels wrong, and one can attribute this to external factors: jobs, girlfriends, etc.

Not knowing any better, I assigned all of my symptoms to other issues, or just didn't know any better and/or figured it was normal. I mean, what's normal anyway and how would you know? It's not like you can jump into a healthy body to gain perspective: "Whoa, hey! No pain. WTF?" In the case of poor memory, I had, of course, the family story of absentmindedness. For the depression, I blamed it on the break-up with my puppy-love girlfriend, or later, just life as a teenager.

In the case of the knee, while I was working with a Rolfer in Maryland, my right tibia suddenly moved back into place on its own, and I immediately remembered a water-skiing accident back in the summer of '79 before the first kneecap dislocation when both skis hit both shins so hard I had a bruise on each of them for three weeks. It turns out the right tibia got knocked out of place, destabilizing the knee above it. So, I thought that was the root cause, but not quite.

After the Lyme died, I got a series of injections to help rebuild the cartilage, a concoction of ozone combined with an agent to encourage regrowth. But Dr. Billica said he believed the root cause behind the knee issue was actually a foot problem, something I'd never considered before, and he referred me to a fellow up in Laramie.

Now, I knew my mother had to wear orthotics; she has what she called the "Lund toe," inherited from her father's side of the family. But despite the fact that all of my life my feet hurt whenever I stood for any period of time, or that I didn't like to hike but instead preferred a slow jog, it never occurred to me that I had the same problem. DOH!

So after a trip to the foot doc and wearing orthotics now for several months, I can say for certain this was the root cause behind the knee, as my stride is longer, my legs are straightening out, and my movements come easier. The waterskiing accident turned out just to be a big trigger, as without the foot problem, I think maybe the leg would have been straighter, and the tibia might well have taken the impact just fine and maybe even snapped back into the correct position on its own. But who knows? You should know that Lyme, as it is happy to do, targets weaknesses in the body. In my case it made things much worse (more arthritic) in the knee through the years.

Lyme also tends to suppress dopamine levels, so one doesn't get much pleasure out of things, the result being a tendency to turn to drugs or alcohol for an artificial high. I got into smoking dope early, and continued on through college, and even took some hallucinogens (LSD, mushrooms), looking for that elusive high that I struggled to get naturally, and as well to escape into my own little world. Both were and are very bad ideas, and I paid a steep price. It took me a boatload of work over the years and a ton of expert help to get the drugs out of my system, heal my brain, repair and calm my nervous system, and deal with the psychological damage.

Probably the worst part about Lyme is chronic fatigue. My friend (with two to three times the number of infections as I had) says the effect of the fatigue is like having a hundred dollars to spend every week in your bank account, while everyone else has a thousand. You end up running a deficit in no time, feeling exhausted and like total crap, until you are forced to back off and allow the coffers to refill. For some, the effects are so strong they end up in bed nearly all day, every day, unable to function.

I think this explains much of my inability to sustain any kind of serious effort over a long time - I just drained the coffers and hit a wall. And I've never been able to do without sleep. If I stayed up late writing a paper for class, I paid for it. A week of this kind of behavior would trash me, completely.

I think my attraction to esoteric martial arts starting in the mid-'80s was in part because I was looking for help of some kind - a lifeline, as my Sifu calls it, and it did work. By my late twenties, my legs were quite strong, and I even went out and won a tennis tournament after only two weeks of practice. It is true that all of the good players were absent that year, so there wasn't much really tough competition, but it gives you an idea of my level of fitness.

Still, I remember training for long-distance runs in my late thirties, but I could never get past a 10k and never could figure out why. Again, I believe now it was because the batteries had little power to spare, given that most of the energy was being used towards the constant fight against a major invasion of bad guys. Tennis is short sprints around the court, and there's time between points to recover. Running, well not so much.

For a while I was looking for an easy fix. I pursued some get-rich-quick schemes, which only work for maybe one person in a million, and other ideas to make life easier and allow more time for rest. Deep down inside I was really hoping just to take time off to sleep in and catch up. I don't think this was really a conscious goal, but an instinct due to that lingering feeling of something being horribly off.

I even pursued becoming a high school English teacher, to the point of almost finishing a master's, for the main purpose of having the summers off, but when I got into the school I realized it wasn't going to work: I didn't have the stamina, and Lord knows I didn't have the right attitude. Something needed fixing, I just didn't know what.

Oh, and some self-inflicted fun that added to my health issues… Back in high school, playing around in a friend's backyard one day, I was being an idiot and as a joke was holding a match to something quite flammable, so in order to prevent this catastrophe, my buddy shot me in the right ring finger with a BB gun. It hurt like an SOB, but I deserved it.

Well, my parents were very anti-gun and I didn't want to make a scene, so I ended up waiting until college to get it taken out. When the BB was removed it was about half its original size. My body had absorbed the rest, and I ended up with a severe case of copper poisoning. Doh! I'm still working on getting all of that out. Too much copper creates almost psychotic responses at different times, depression, and all kinds of weird emotional responses. Already having Lyme, this just amplified some of my weird anti-social behavior.

I knew none of this when I got married to the wrong woman in my mid-forties. She was in the relationship for herself, as it turned out, and this severely drained my energy (and my bank account), to the point when seven years in, I just couldn't take it anymore and broke it off. Doing so I probably saved my own life, as I'm pretty sure I was heading smack dab for a heart attack. My health was pretty much touch and go for a long time after that.

Thank God for my martial arts school, which I rejoined a couple of years later. I am very blessed indeed, with great friends, to be back where I belong, doing what I know I should be doing, heading in the direction I need to go, and doing what I love, like writing this book.

Yeah, it's all been worth it, and then some. Hard to believe, I know, but I actually wouldn't change any of it. I think I had some hard lessons to learn in this lifetime: how to work hard, be persistent, be a good friend, and be selfless and grateful for all life has to offer.

Chapter Thirteen - Whakatane and White Island

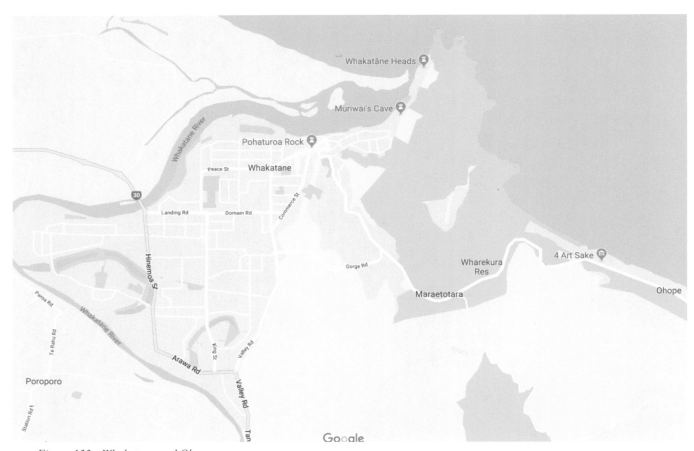

Figure 133 - Whakatane and Ohope

Back in Whakatane, I pulled back on my exercising to just some rides around town, and even started running. At that point my knee still didn't go down hills or stairs too well—I sort of had a hitch—but I could get by. I could easily run for an hour, though, and did so among the hills that guard the town, and even discovered the remains of an old Maori fort: it had a great view in all directions and was perfectly positioned for defense.

There's an old trail that runs eastward from the town, up and down over various hills, with lots of steps—steep steps at times. The first part is quite private, with very few people. It leads you through woods of varying design (oaks, maples, and pine), to rainforest, to farmland, and back again. It even runs along Ohope Beach at one point. Ohope has a gentle slope with a few quiet motels and houses situated back and across a frontage road, allowing the sandy regions to remain public.

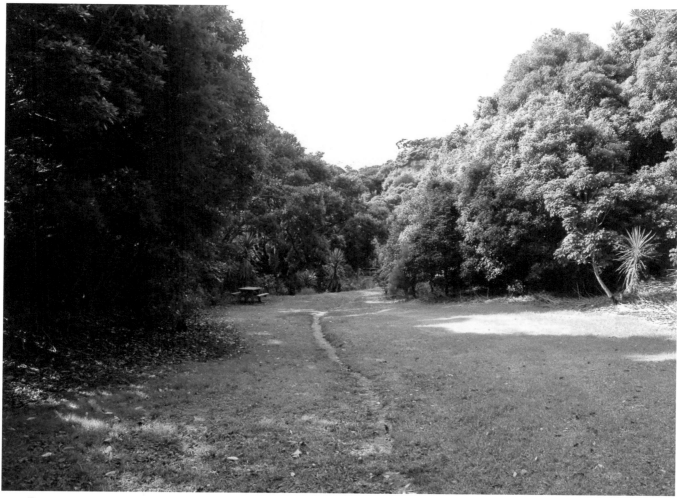

Figure 134 - Paths in the hills to the east above Whakatane

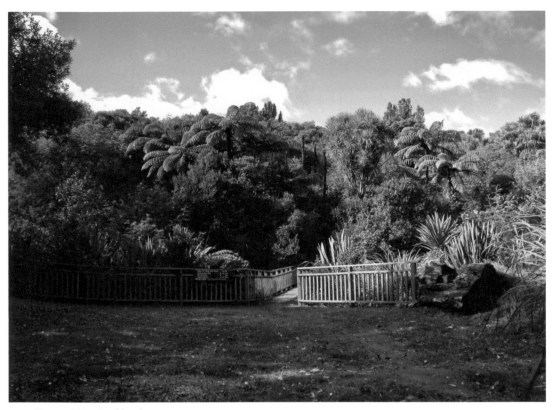

Figure 135 - Parkland

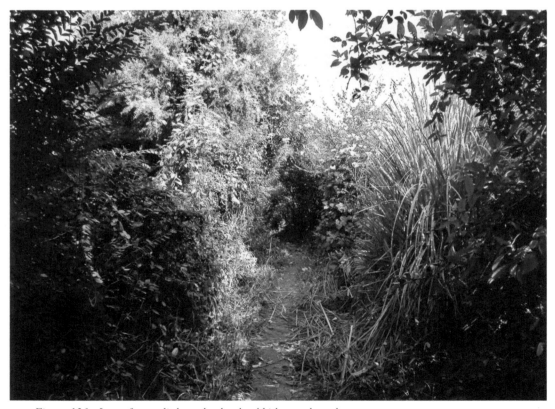

Figure 136 - Lots of great little paths that lead hither and yonder

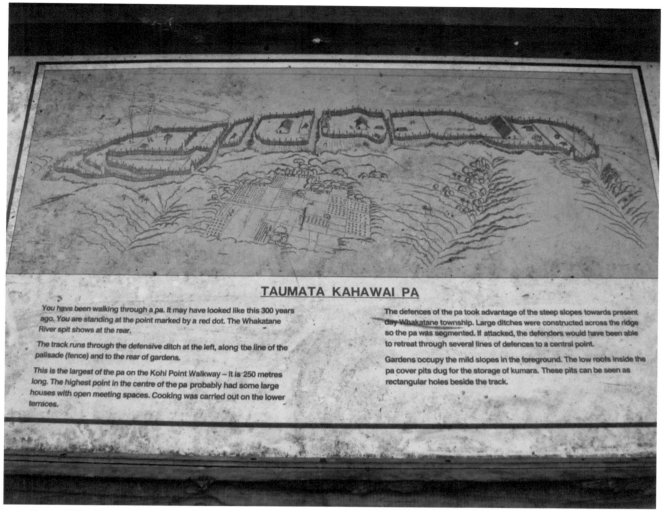

Figure 137 - Plaque of the old Maori fort

The text of the plaque goes as follows: "You have been walking through a pa. It may have looked like this 300 years ago. You are standing at the point marked by a red dot. The Whakatane River spit shows at the rear. The track runs through the defensive ditch at the left, along the line of the palisade (fence) and to the rear of gardens. This is the largest of the pa on the Kohi Point Walkway - it is 250 meters long. The highest point in the centre of the pa probably had some large houses with open meeting spaces. Cooking was carried out on the lower terraces. The defense of the pa took advantage of the steep slopes towards present day Whakatane township. Large ditches were constructed across the ridge, so the pa was segmented. If attacked, the defenders would have been able to retreat through several lines of defenses to a central point. Gardens occupy the mild slopes in the foreground. The low roots inside the pa cover pits dug for the storage of kimora. These pits can be seen as rectangular holes beside the track."

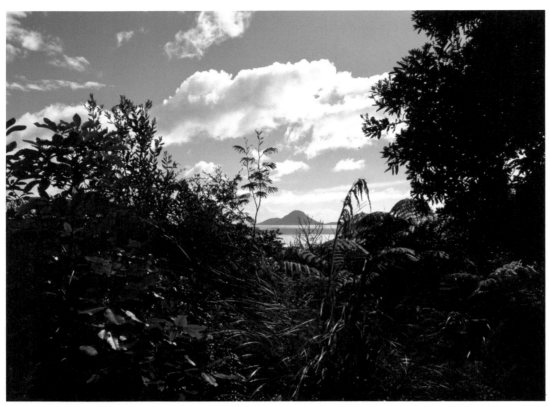

Figure 138 - From the trail looking at White Island

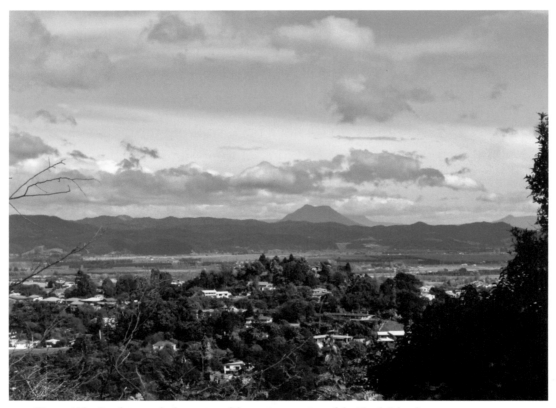

Figure 139 - South towards the center of the eastern section of the North Island

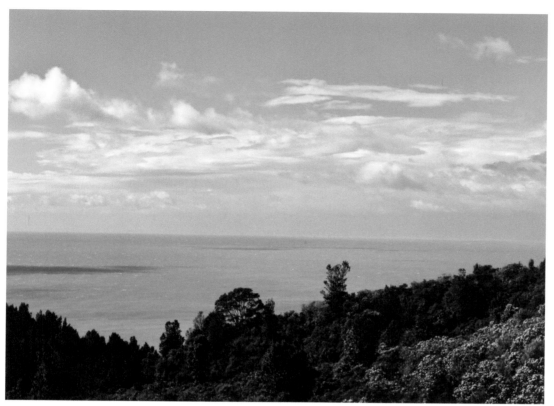

Figure 140 - Tasman Bay

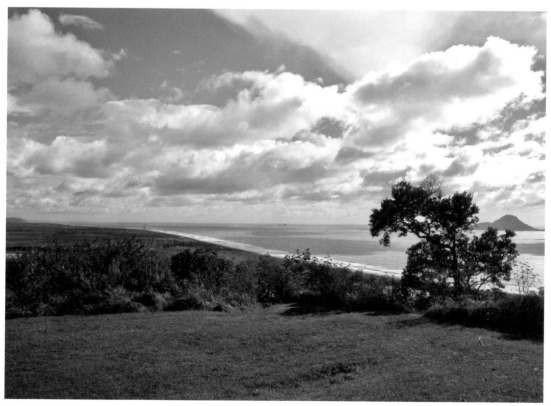

Figure 141 - A view back west

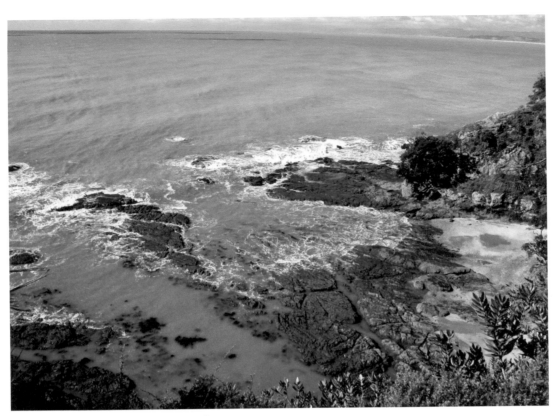

Figure 142 - Towards Ohope Beach

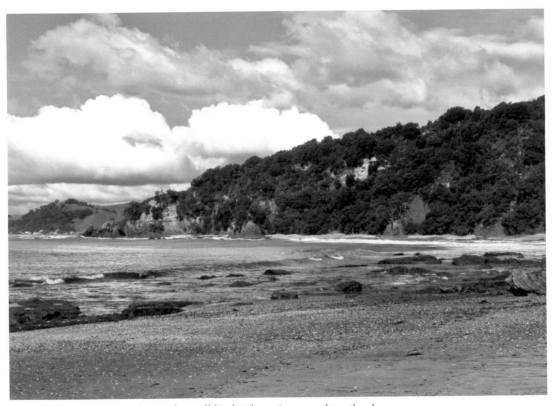

Figure 143 - The trail runs along all kinds of terrain, even along the shore

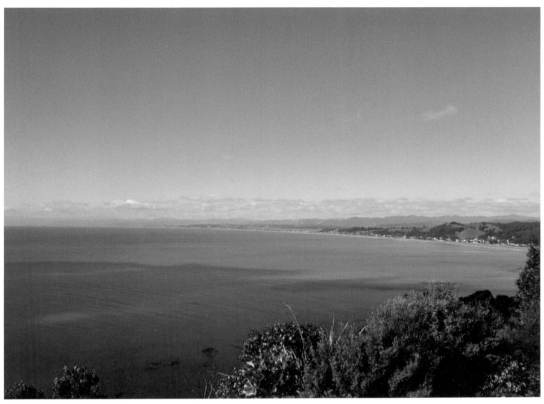

Figure 144 - More of the beautiful Tasman Bay

Figure 145 - Somewhere in that direction is Fiji

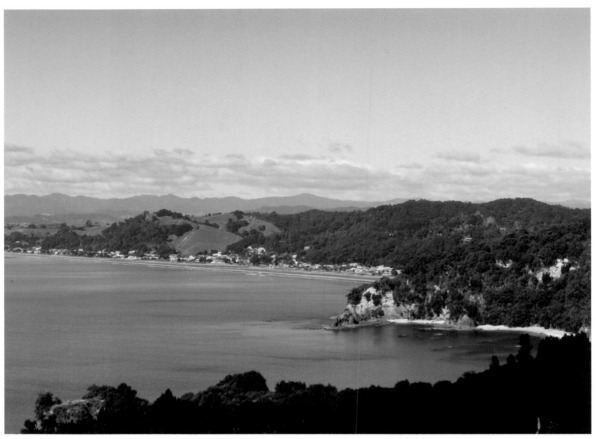

Figure 146 - Ohope Beach in the distance

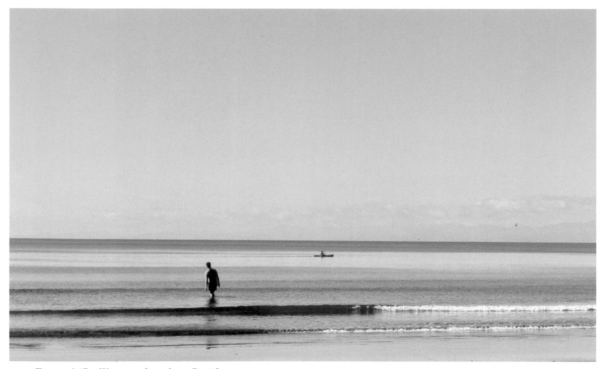

Figure 147 - Warm, salty, clean Pacific waters

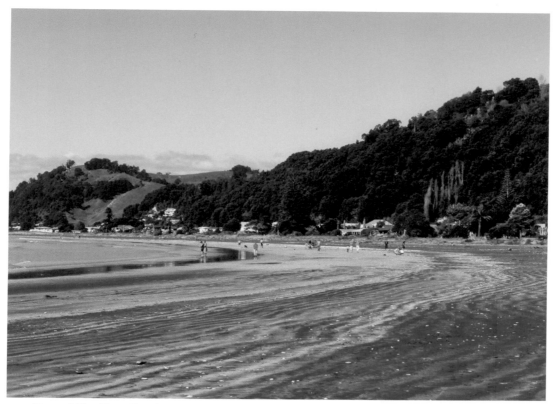

Figure 148 - Ohope Beach

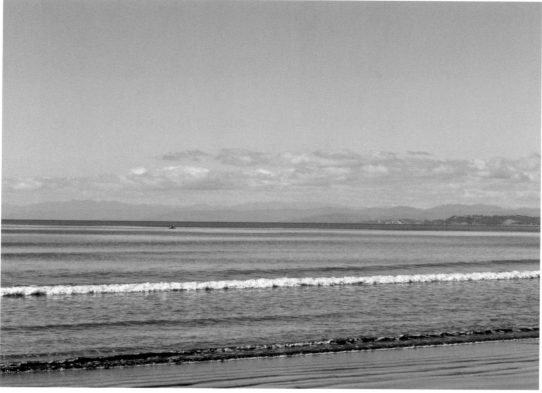

Figure 149 - More of the beach, looking east

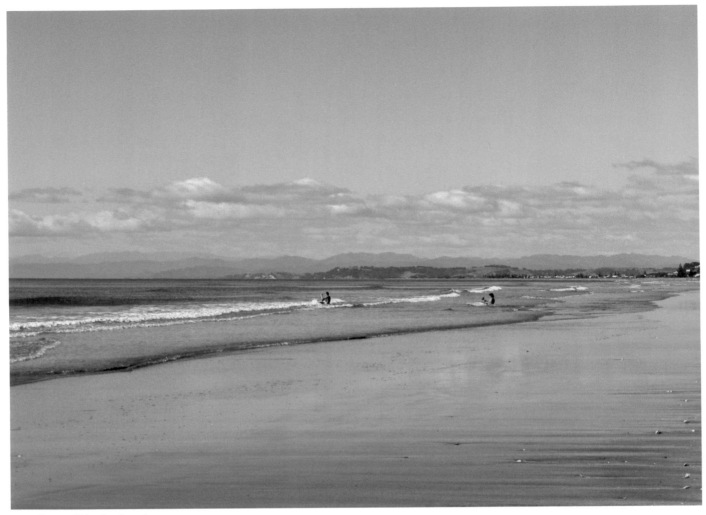

Figure 150 - Sea kayaks

My room in Whakatane was only NW$30 a night, and on the morning of the White Island tour, I enjoyed the best breakfast I'd ever had up to then, or since! Due to New Zealand being quite remote, they had developed the farm-to-table idea out of necessity. So the big mushroom was fresh, the eggs right from the farm, the sausage the same; there was homemade wheat toast, and the potatoes . . . oooh la la. With the volcanic run-off fertilizing the eastern farmland, it made for naturally mineral-rich food that tasted just wonderful.

I took a few rides around the town, but really, I was done. I think I stayed a total of two weeks there before a friend called with a job offer (my mentor, looking out for me, bless him), and since I was burned out on riding and running low on cash, I decided it was about time to leave.

As for the tour of the White Island volcano, it's a two-hour ride out, with lots of their version of a dolphin, along with something bigger lurking nearby. The island had a little factory that mined sulfur at one point, but toxic clouds from the occasional burp cause health problems and eventually they quit. It was an interesting walk around the caldera with nothing spectacular: no lava flows or anything like that. Quite calm indeed.

I was talking with a young lady one day in the hotel lounge, and it turned out she was going diving off this island. Apparently about sixty feet down there are all kinds of vents and weird undersea flora and fauna.

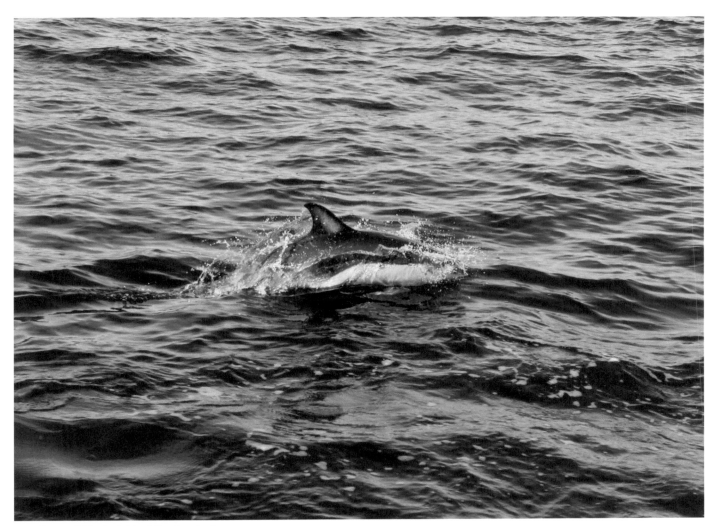

Figure 151 - Dolphin following the boat

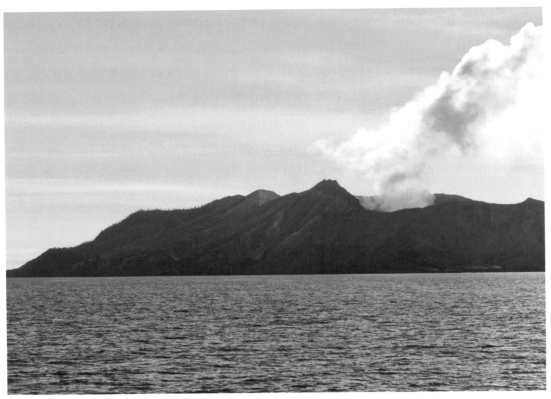

Figure 152 - Towards White Island

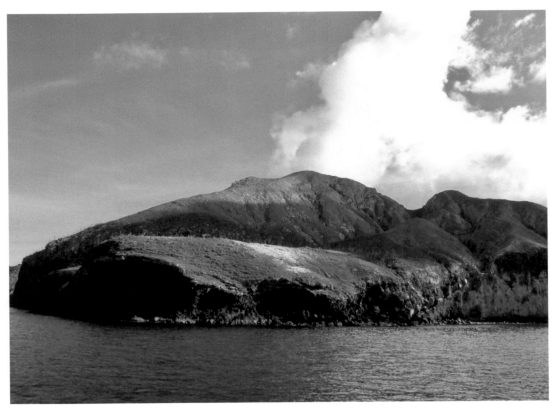

Figure 153 - Scary looking caves - good hiding places for the creatures of Dr. Moreau

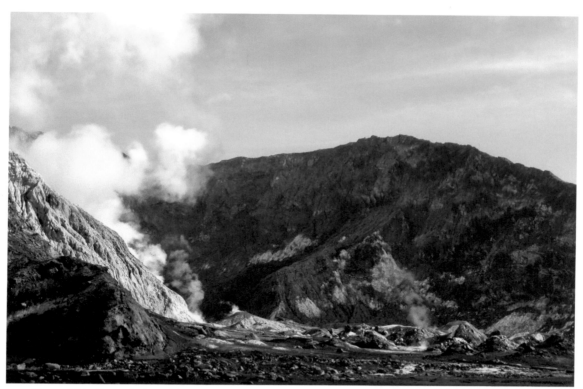

Figure 154 - Towards the caldera

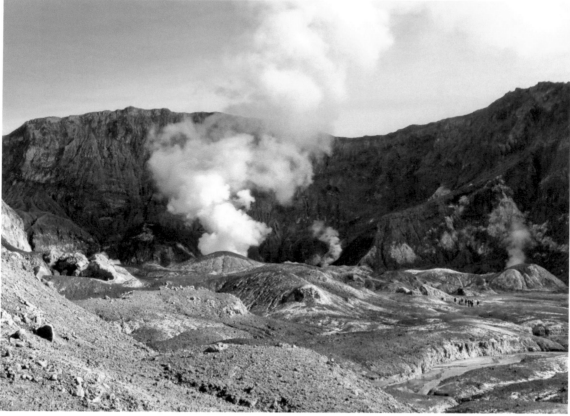

Figure 155 - Mars, is it?

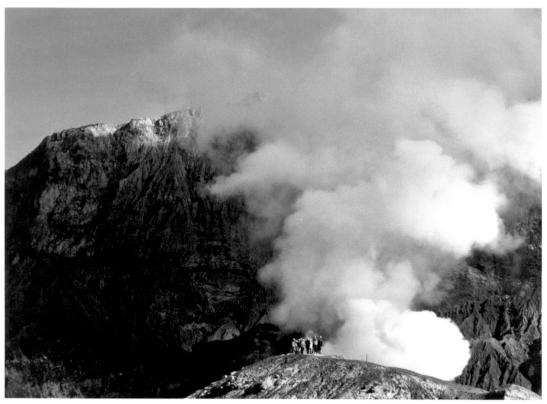

Figure 156 - For size perspective

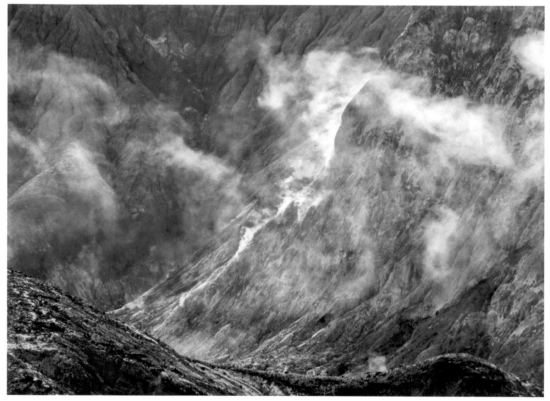

Figure 157 - Strange reddish moss, yellow sulphuric gasses, and other fun

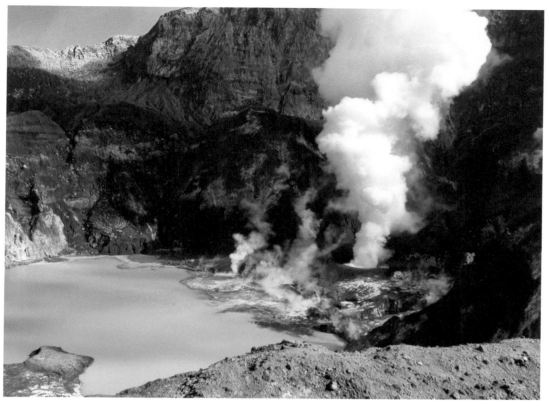

Figure 158 - Shall we go for a swim, dear? You first!

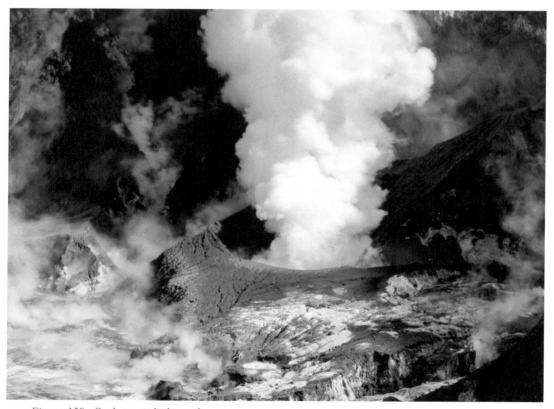

Figure 159 - Such a cute little...volcano

141

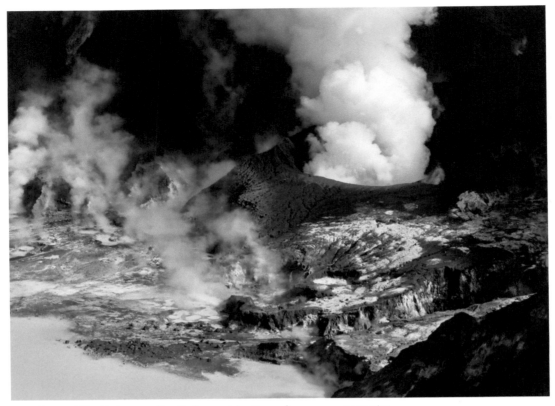

Figure 160 - No lava, sadly. Or fortunately. Depends on your perspective.

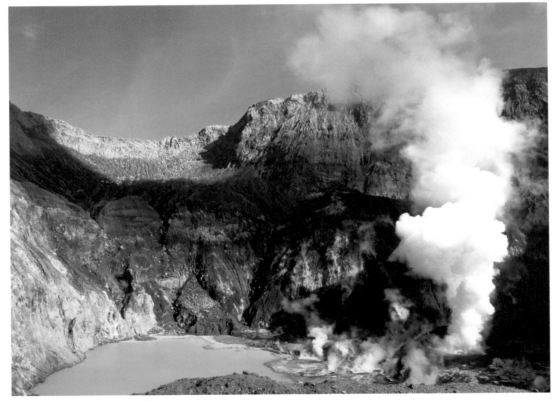

Figure 161 - Huge walls surrounding the cone

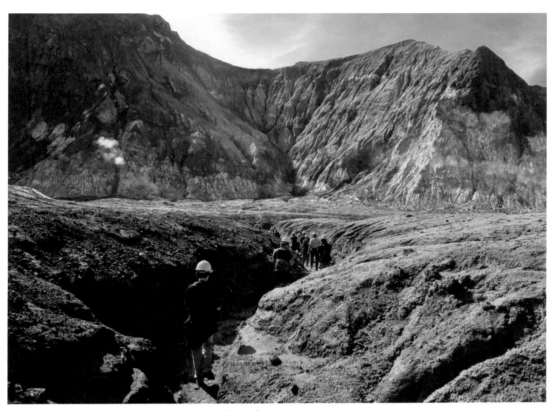

Figure 162 - A walkway through the old lava flows

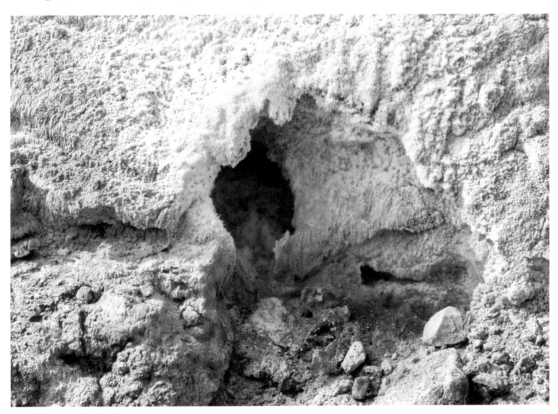

Figure 163 - Sulfur vent

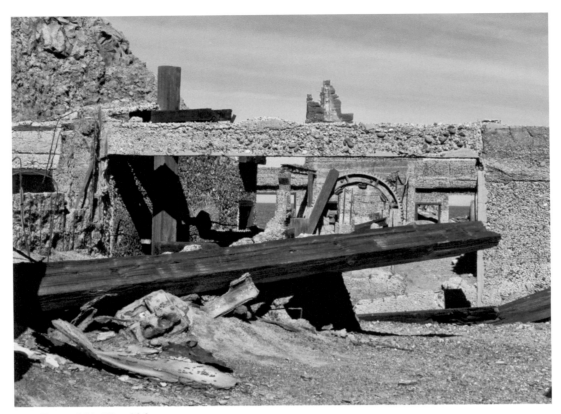

Figure 164 - The old factory

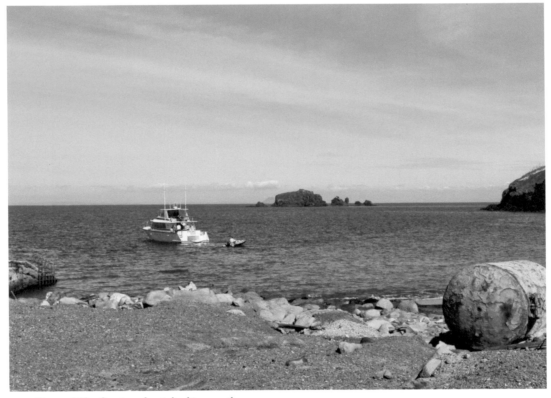

Figure 165 - Our tour boat, looking south

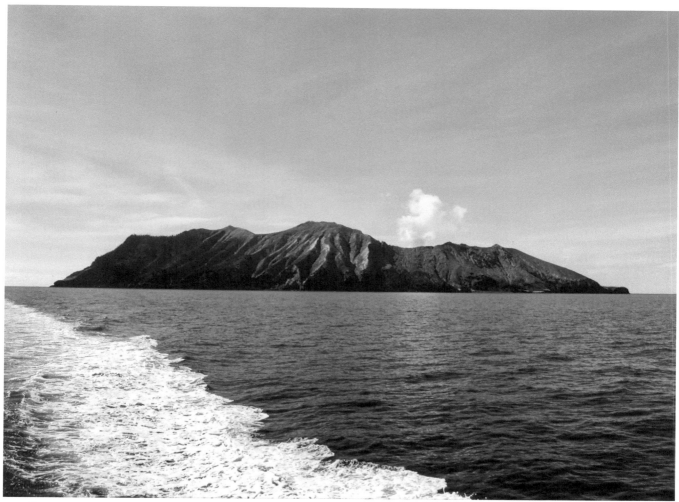

Figure 166 - One last look before we say goodbye

A few days later I took the bus back to Auckland and caught a flight out on a Tuesday, late. It was the middle of May, 2002. I had been sick for thirty-four years and didn't even know it, but it would be another sixteen before I really started making progress down the long road back to health.

Epilogue

As I write this in the summer of 2019, I'm still on the road to recovery, and probably will be for another year. My brain is working better; it's been slow going but the fog is lifting, and I can concentrate for longer periods of time. Mornings can be rough, however. I no longer have "those days" when I'm totally trashed and sitting on the couch is about all I can do. Instead, I can get some work done, and move my life forward.

My body still has a lot to deal with, however. My balance is kind of whacky, as my feet adjust to the orthotics and my foundation continues to shift and adjust. My knee is getting more support but is far from okay. I'm not sure what the future holds there - I may always have some arthritis. My large intestine is working well, but my lungs still have a lot of room for improvement. My heart is strong, and the kidneys (the batteries of the body) continue to recover. My liver still struggles to get rid of left-over toxins, but I'm not a drinker and I eat clean, so that much is good. Blood sugar is fine - I was pre-diabetic after my marriage, but I'm fine now, (though I still avoid candy and sodas like the plague), and my blood pressure is spot on.

For those of you still struggling, keep the faith! I firmly believe somewhere; somebody has a solution for your ills. Call Dr. Billica - maybe he can help, and if he can't, he'll say so and refer you to someone else who can. Healing is a personal journey, and it takes a lot of suffering, a ton of hard work, and the will and persistence to get there, but it's worth it, and you may find you're a very different person in the end.

About the Author

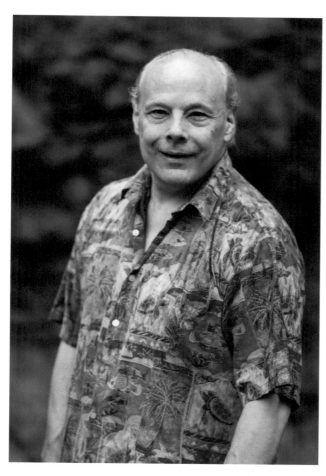

Mr. Main was born in California, raised in New York, spent summers in Maine, lived for a number of years in Virginia and Colorado, and currently resides in Wyoming. He received his B.A. in English from the University of Colorado at Boulder, his M.S. in Technology Management from George Mason University, and is an information assurance and cybersecurity professional with over twenty-four years of experience.

Before this career, Mr. Main worked in all kinds of different jobs, from washing dishes, to taxi cab driver, to carpentry and landscaping, and even co-owned a bridal boutique with his ex in Fairfax, Virginia called Maria's Bridal Designs.

Mr. Main has written poetry, short stories, songs, and is currently working on the final edits of a science fiction novel.

CPSIA information can be obtained
at www.ICGtesting.com
Printed in the USA
BVHW021159290819
557142BV00005B/30/P